# THE
# PET LOVER'S
# GUIDE TO
# CANINE ARTHRITIS
# & JOINT PROBLEMS

# About The Pet Lover's Guide Series

**Y**our pets are important members of your family. When they have a medical condition, you want them to get the best care that can be provided. You also want to know everything you can about their condition, including all the treatment options. This series, written by leading veterinary authors, will help you, as a pet owner, understand the causes, diagnosis, treatment, and prevention options for many common conditions your pets may have.

This series provides quality veterinary information, written by the veterinary leaders your veterinarian trusts, but in an easy-to understand manner that allows you to talk with your veterinarian about your pet's condition. **The books in this series are not intended as substitutes for visits to your veterinarian.** Instead, they should be read as a way to get more information about your pet's condition so that you'll know what to do, what to ask, and what to expect when you take your pet to your veterinarian.

# THE
# PET LOVER'S GUIDE TO CANINE ARTHRITIS & JOINT PROBLEMS

## Kurt Schulz, DVM, DACVS

Associate Professor
School of Veterinary Medicine
University of California, Davis;
Animal Medical Center of New England
Nashua, New Hampshire

**Brian Beale, DVM, DACVS**
Gulf Coast Veterinary Specialists
Houston, Texas

**Ian Holsworth, BVSc, DACVS**
Veterinary Medical and
Surgical Group
Ventura, California

**Sandra L. Hudson, MBA, CCRP**
Canine Rehabilitation and
Conditioning Center
Round Rock, Texas;
Adjunct Professor
Texas A & M University
College Station, Texas

**Don Hulse, DVM, DACVS**
Professor
College of Veterinary Medicine
Texas A & M University
College Station, Texas

*With a contribution from*
**Autumn P. Davidson DVM, MS, DACVIM**
Adjunct Professor, School of Veterinary Medicine
University of California, Davis;
Animal Care Center of Sonoma
Rohnert Park, California

SAUNDERS
ELSEVIER

# ELSEVIER
# SAUNDERS

11830 Westline Industrial Drive
St. Louis, Missouri 63146

ISBN 13: 978-1-4160-2614-3
ISBN 10: 1-4160-2614-2

**The Pet Lover's Guide to Canine Arthritis and
Joint Problems**
Copyright © 2006, Elsevier Inc.

---

### Notice

Neither the Publisher nor the Authors assume any responsibility for any loss or injury
and/or damage to persons or property arising out of or related to any use of the material contained in this book. It is the responsibility of the treating practitioner, relying on
independent expertise and knowledge of the patient, to determine the best treatment
and method of application for the patient.

---

The Publisher

ISBN 13: 978-1-4160-2614-3
ISBN 10: 1-4160-2614-2

*Publishing Director:* Linda Duncan
*Senior Editor:* Liz Fathman
*Developmental Editor:* Shelly Stringer
*Publishing Services Manager:* Patricia Tannian
*Project Manager:* John Casey
*Cover/Book Design Direction:* Amy Buxton
*Cover/Book Design:* Bill Smith Studio

Printed in United States of America

Last digit is the print number:   9   8   7   6   5   4   3   2   1

For my parents, Joan and Allan, for their
never ending support
**KS**

For my children, Jared, Danielle, and Isabel
**BB**

For my children, Grace and Will
**IGH**

For my husband, Don
**SH**

For my parents, Charles and Martha
**DH**

To our clients

for their dedication to the

health and happiness

of their canine companions

# Foreword

There was a time when the diagnosis of osteoarthritis meant the beginning of progressive incapacity for our canine companions. However, in the past two decades, new scientific advances on several fronts have dramatically changed this likelihood of inevitable, unstoppable decline to one of hope, continued activity, and pain-free living. A better understanding of the preexisting conditions that cause osteoarthritis, improved techniques for joint imaging, and better methods of evaluating joint movement have all improved the ability of veterinarians to diagnose joint problems earlier and successfully treat them for longer periods of time. Also, more medications for relieving the pain of arthritis have been tested and approved for use in the past 10 to 15 years. In addition, as we continue to refine the various surgeries for joint replacement and for cruciate ligament repairs, we increasingly provide hope for long-term athletic joint function for thousands of our pets each year.

Despite the explosion of knowledge and advancements in the diagnosis and treatment of osteoarthritis in both humans and companion animals, there has been very little reliable and easily understood information written for the companion pet owner. Much of the information available for the concerned owner is incomplete, contradictory or even misleading. This problem has only been magnified by the Internet and the wealth of available information it contains. This book bridges the gap between academic knowledge about osteoarthritis in our pets and the practical application of those treatment principles and options that are currently available to the veterinarian and pet owner. Written by a group of leading experts in the field of veterinary orthopedics, *The Pet Lover's Guide to Canine Arthritis and Joint Problems* is a necessary addition to every dog owner's library. The authors, lead by Dr. Kurt Schulz, have created a book that addresses all aspects of this common disease. This book is a complete and readable source of information about osteoarthritis that does not shy away from any of the tough issues currently facing pet owners when trying to treat their ailing canine companions. For the reader looking for answers to questions about diagnosis or possible treatments, whether they are conventional or controversial, this book provides essential, concise, easily understandable facts and generally agreed-upon professional opinions of veterinary specialists that will help every owner to be better informed.

*American College of Veterinary Surgeons*

# The American College of Veterinary Surgeons

The American College of Veterinary Surgeons (ACVS) was founded in 1965 as a nonprofit educational and certifying organization with 35 professional veterinary surgeons as charter members. Today, the College is approximately 1150 members strong with members participating in diverse career areas including private and academic clinical practice, administration, industry, and government. ACVS surgeons treat a broad range of species, including companion animals such as dogs and cats, as well as birds, wildlife, zoo animals, food-producing animals, and horses.

The goals of the ACVS are to advance the art and science of veterinary surgery for the benefit of all animal species. The ACVS has developed programs that provide rigorous postdoctoral residency programs in veterinary surgery. Veterinarians are certified through documentation of supervised training and examination as specialists in surgery, and members are encouraged to pursue and report original investigations to advance the collective body of surgical knowledge. Members of the College are called Diplomates and have devoted at least 4 years to advanced clinical training in surgery under the supervision of other Diplomates, passed a certifying examination, and published at least one original article in the veterinary literature.

The official seal of the ACVS symbolizes the ancient origin of surgery in both animals and man. The centaur is Chiron, who was known for his wisdom and justice. Chiron taught surgery and medicine in his school to such famous pupils as Apollo, Jason, and Achilles. The ACVS seal can be displayed only by Diplomates of the College or with special permission of the college. The presence of the ACVS seal indicates endorsement by the ACVS of the quality and scholarly presentation of the contents.

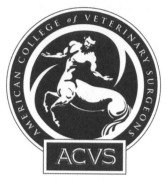

# Acknowledgments

The content of this book is the result of the contributions of numerous surgeons, residents, and technicians who have over the years worked to develop better ways to help owners help their pets. The original concept is a culmination of the materials we have prepared for our clients to educate them on the orthopedic health of their dogs. The format was inspired by other publications designed to communicate complex topics to individuals without education in the field. The layout and style are designed to be both fun and educational. The result is a book that is first in its kind in the pet health care field and whose format has been adapted to an entire series of pet health care books. Our ultimate goal is to educate and assist in optimizing the health and quality of life of our patients and their owners.

Special thanks are due to Steve Budsberg for his tremendous objective knowledge of NSAIDs, Robert Taylor for his support through the ACVS, John Doval for his incredible talent in graphics, Steve Fox for his long-term support in this project, Daryl Millis, Jackie Woelz, and David Levine for assistance with the physical therapy section, Phil Roudebush, Barry Watson, Melody Raasch, Denise Elliott, Andrea Fascetti, Stefanie Oppenheim, Dottie Laflamme, Scott J. Campbell, Sean Delaney, William Burkholder, Robert Armstrong, and Barbara Eves for technical guidance in nutrition, NSAIDs, and supplementation, Herbert Addison for editorial guidance, Liz Fathman for pursuing the idea, and, of course, to Shelly "crack the whip" Stringer for keeping us on track.

# Introduction

Perhaps you have just taken your young dog to your veterinarian and were told that she has a disease that will lead to arthritis in the future. Or perhaps you have an older dog that has experienced increasing reluctance to exercise and shows more stiffness or lameness. In either situation, a diagnosis of arthritis can be extremely concerning to dog owners. Besides the main concern for your dog's welfare, there are questions about the safety of treatments, conflicting information, and cost.

Dog owners want nothing more for their pets than for them to be well and happy. When your dog has arthritis, you want to help him feel better. While osteoarthritis in most cases cannot be cured, with your veterinarian's help the pain and disability of osteoarthritis can be dramatically lessened.

The purpose of this book is to help you understand the causes and treatments of osteoarthritis in dogs. We have attempted to write this book based on sound scientific evidence and experience. In situations where we have strong opinions regarding therapies, they have been clearly titled as Where We Stand.

## What Is Osteoarthritis?

Osteoarthritis (OA) is one of the most frequent causes of physical disability in adult dogs. Osteoarthritis is a joint disease that mostly affects the articular cartilage. Articular cartilage is the slippery tissue that covers the ends of bones in a joint. Healthy cartilage allows bones to glide over one another. It also absorbs energy from the shock of physical movement. In osteoarthritis, the surface layer of cartilage breaks down and wears away. This allows bones under the cartilage to rub together, causing pain, swelling, and loss of motion of the joint. Our clinical experience suggest that 20 percent of middle aged and

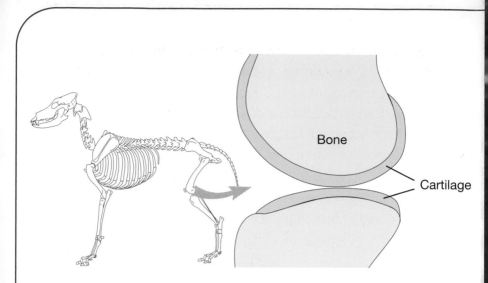

Bone

Cartilage

as much as 90 percent of elderly dogs have one or more joints affected by osteoarthritis. The result is joint pain, limited movement, and alteration of lifestyle. Some lifestyle changes that often seem to go with the discomfort of osteoarthritis include depression, aggressive behavior toward family members, reluctance to rise from a lying position, trouble participating in everyday normal activities, and exercise intolerance.

Scientists do not know yet what causes osteoarthritis, but they suspect a combination of factors, including being overweight, the aging process, joint injury, stresses on the joints from certain sports activities, and perhaps a sedentary lifestyle. Despite these challenges, most dogs with osteoarthritis can lead active and happy lives. Success depends on an accurate diagnosis from your veterinarian and the use of multimodal (more than one method) treatment strategies.

We sincerely hope that this book will help you work with your veterinarian or veterinary orthopedic surgeon to make the most of your dog's quality of life. We feel strongly that with continued scientific progress, the outlook for dogs with osteoarthritis is bright.

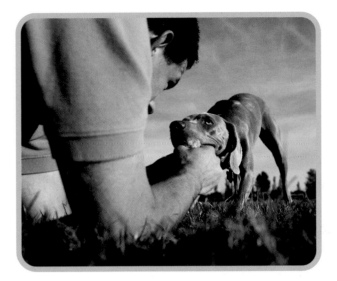

# Contents

# PART ONE

# Osteoarthritis in Your Dog

CHAPTER **1**

# WHAT IS OSTEOARTHRITIS?

In this chapter we look at the normal structures of your dog's joints and the changes they go through when your dog has osteoarthritis.

Many terms are used to describe the condition of osteoarthritis: "arthritis," "osteoarthritis," and "degenerative joint disease." But whichever name is used, one thing that can be agreed on is that osteoarthritis is a painful disease that limits a dog's ability to move and function normally.

The normal joint is made up of bone, cartilage, and the soft tissue that surrounds the joint, including ligaments, tendons, and joint capsule. Each of these structures changes when your dog has osteoarthritis, causing the pain and loss of function that are the hallmarks of this disease.

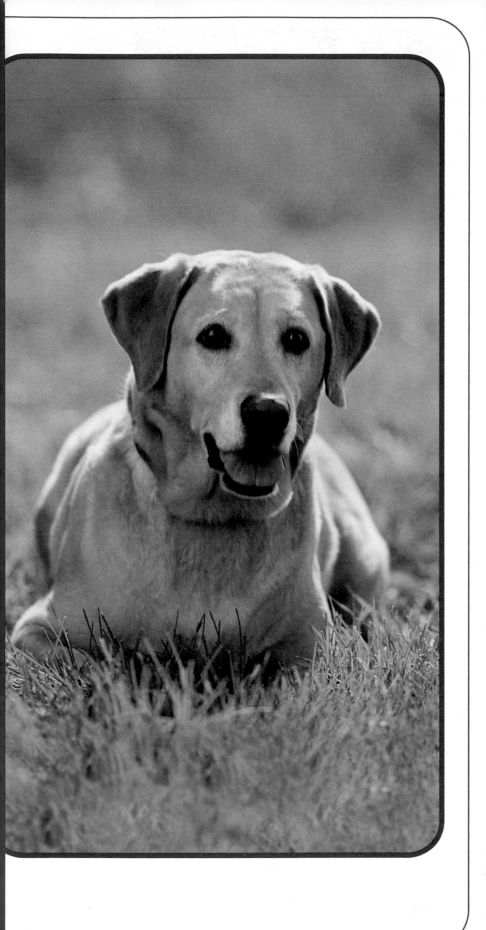

# The Normal Joint

The function of joints is to permit movement and support the body. To do this, joints are made of:

- **Soft tissue**
- **Hard tissue**
- **Joint fluid**

## Soft Tissues

Soft tissues are made up of the ligaments, the joint capsule that surrounds a joint, and the muscle-tendon units (where muscle attaches to bone). The ligaments hold the joint in place and control joint movement. For example, the **cruciate ligaments** in your dog's knee joint prevent the bones of the knee joint from sliding backward and forward when the knee joint moves. Sprained or torn ligaments allow the joint to move too much or incorrectly, which leads to grinding and damaging of the cartilage. The result of this cartilage damage is osteoarthritis. Ligament damage also causes joint pain by allowing the surrounding soft tissues to stretch and tear.

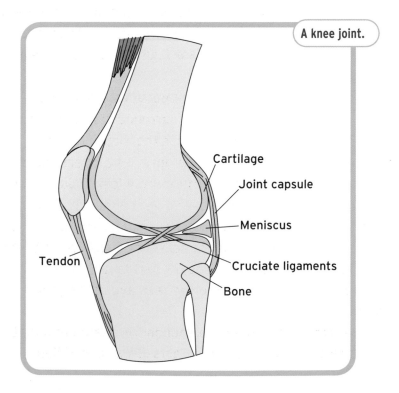

A knee joint.

Cartilage

Joint capsule

Meniscus

Tendon

Cruciate ligaments

Bone

Another type of soft tissue surrounding the joint is the joint capsule. This capsule has two layers: a strong outer layer and an inner layer. The cells lining the inner layer of the joint capsule produce a thick fluid called **synovial fluid** that lubricates the joint and feeds the cartilage. The joint capsule also affects the joint's immune functions. The joint capsule has an excellent blood supply and nerve supply—two factors that have a big effect on arthritis pain.

Muscle-tendon units are the third soft tissue in a joint. These are the points where tendons attach to bone and often are located very close to joints. Some muscle-tendon units in the body hold joints in place and keep them from moving incorrectly, for example, in the "rotator cuff" (the muscles surrounding the shoulder joint). Because they are located so close to the joint, when the joint is injured, the muscle-tendon units can be damaged as well. This damage results in muscle pain when the joint is moved.

## Hard Tissues

Cartilage and the bone underneath it make up the hard tissues of the joint. Cartilage has two jobs: to absorb shock and to minimize the joint's surface friction to ease and improve movement.

Cartilage is made up of three parts: cartilage cells (**chondrocytes**), a **matrix** that surrounds the cells, and water. The cartilage cells produce the matrix that surrounds them. Cartilage cells do not have a direct blood supply, so they get their nutrition from joint fluid. As a result, cartilage cells do not have a very good nutritional supply. One of the reasons why it is difficult for cartilage to heal is that instead of a direct blood supply right to the cartilage, the joint fluid feeds the cartilage nutrients. These nutrients are fed into the cartilage as the joint moves.

The **cartilage matrix** is a sponge-like scaffolding that gives cartilage its structure. It acts like a water-filled

3

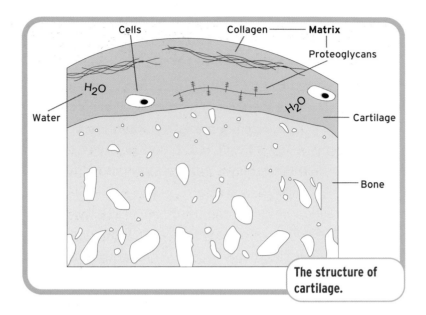

Cells — Collagen —— **Matrix**

Proteoglycans

$H_2O$

$H_2O$

Water

Cartilage

Bone

The structure of cartilage.

shock absorber, squeezing out water when it is under high pressure and absorbing water when it is under low pressure. This in-and-out movement of water lets the cartilage absorb shocks to the joints as your dog moves, and it also carries nutrients throughout the cartilage to the cartilage cells. The cartilage surface is smooth, with low friction, allowing joints to move freely.

The cartilage matrix acts like a water-filled shock absorber, squeezing out water under high pressure and absorbing water under low pressure.

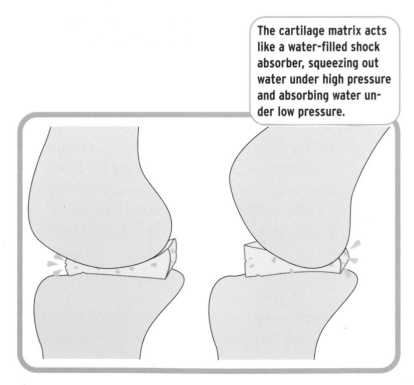

# The Cartilage Matrix

The cartilage matrix is made up of a combination of chemical substances, the two most important of which are **collagen** and **proteoglycans**.

Collagen is found in practically all tissues in the body. It provides strength to tissues, and it helps protect cartilage from tearing and breaking down due to normal activity or injury. Think of collagen as strands of rope that give strength to body tissues.

Proteoglycans attract water to the matrix. The well-hydrated matrix provides the important "shock absorber" effect of cartilage. These proteoglycans are formed by a hyaluronic acid core attached to many small molecules called **glycosaminoglycans** (GAGs).

Hyaluronic acid also is found in joint fluid and keeps the joint lubricated. Injection of hyaluronic acid into the joint or muscle is a treatment for osteoarthritis.

The most familiar glycosaminoglycan is **chondroitin sulfate**. This molecule is commonly found in nutritional supplements for joint disease.

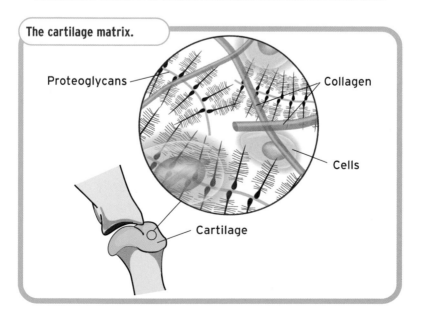

The cartilage matrix.

Proteoglycans

Collagen

Cells

Cartilage

The cartilage matrix is a key area in the treatment of osteoarthritis. Many nutritional supplements used in the treatment of osteoarthritis are based on the content and structure of this matrix.

Bone under the cartilage determines the shape of the cartilage surface. It provides the strength that your dog's joints need to support the tremendous loads placed on them. It also supplies the joint with blood vessels and nerves.

## Joint Fluid

Joint fluid acts as a lubricant for the joint and carries nutrients to the cartilage. It is mostly made of water but also includes important molecules such as **hyaluronic acid** (HA). This HA is the major ingredient in joint fluid that makes the fluid thick and provides lubrication. Injections of HA sometimes are used for short-term pain relief in osteoarthritis.

# The Osteoarthritic Joint

Osteoarthritis causes changes to all of the structures of the normal joint. The basic changes include:

- **Wearing down and cracking of cartilage**
- **Thickening and stiffening of the joint capsule** (fibrosis)
- **Hardening and grinding down of the bone beneath the cartilage** (sclerosis and eburnation)
- **New bone growth around the joint** (osteophytosis)
- **Thinning of joint fluid**

## Cartilage Changes

Osteoarthritis affects your dog's cartilage in different ways. The ability of cartilage to work normally depends on its water content. But osteoarthritis changes the water

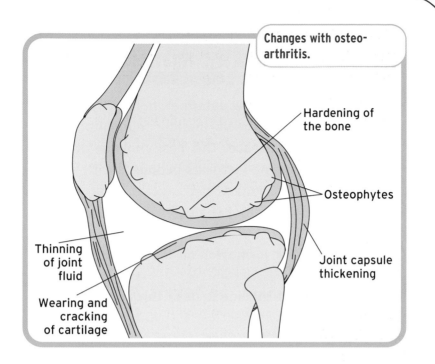

Changes with osteo-arthritis.

Hardening of the bone

Osteophytes

Thinning of joint fluid

Joint capsule thickening

Wearing and cracking of cartilage

content of cartilage. Early in osteoarthritis, cartilage absorbs water and swells up, making it softer and more easily injured. In the middle and late stages of osteoarthritis, the cartilage loses the ability to hold water, causing the cartilage to crack and wear down. When the disease is severe, the cartilage may wear through completely, exposing the bone underneath.

## Joint Capsule Changes

The main changes in the joint capsule caused by osteoarthritis are fibrosis, thickening, and decreased blood supply. Osteoarthritis causes inflammation of the joint capsule, which then leads to decreased blood supply. In tissues that have poor (low) blood supply, fibrous scar tissue forms during healing. Scar tissue in the joint capsule does not work or move as well as the original tissue. Fibrous scar tissue causes arthritic joints to be stiff and less flexible.

## Grading of Osteoarthritis

During surgery your veterinarian may "grade" your dog's osteoarthritis, in order to monitor progression of the disease. The most common grading method for osteoarthritis in dogs is with the modified Outterbridge scale:

- Grade I—softening of the cartilage (chondro-malacia)
- Grade II—fiber formation on the cartilage surface
- Grade III—full-thickness gaps through the cartilage
- Grade IV—full-thickness loss of cartilage
- Grade V—polishing and hardening of the exposed bone (eburnation)

## Bone Changes

The bone beneath the joint surface changes early in osteoarthritis. The bone directly beneath the cartilage becomes harder and more dense (**sclerotic**). At the edge of the joint, small and irregular bumps of new bone (**osteophytes**) often form. These areas of new bone growth do not normally affect joint movement and function, so removing them will probably not help your dog. In fact, osteophytes often grow back rapidly after they are removed if the osteoarthritis continues. Osteophytes are, however, useful in diagnosing osteoarthritis, as they are easy to see on radiographs (x-ray films).

## Joint Fluid Changes

In arthritic joints, the joint fluid is thin and does not lubricate enough for normal joint function. This poor-quality joint fluid is caused by an increased water content in the joint fluid and a decrease in the molecules (like HA) that normally lubricate the joint surfaces.

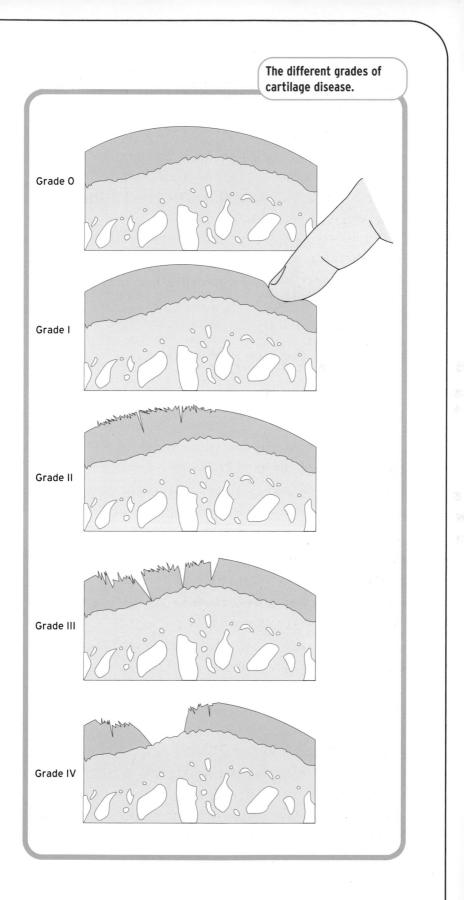

The different grades of cartilage disease.

Grade 0

Grade I

Grade II

Grade III

Grade IV

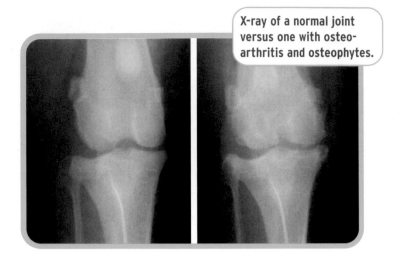

X-ray of a normal joint versus one with osteo-arthritis and osteophytes.

## Cycle of Osteoarthritis

In many cases, osteoarthritis progresses slowly and works against itself to cause more cartilage destruction—a so-called vicious circle: The damage to your dog's un-healthy joint causes inflammation, which causes even more damage to the joint. The osteoarthritis then gets worse and worse and continues in a similar downward spi-ral. The fact that the joint cartilage has a limited ability to heal contributes to this downward cycle.

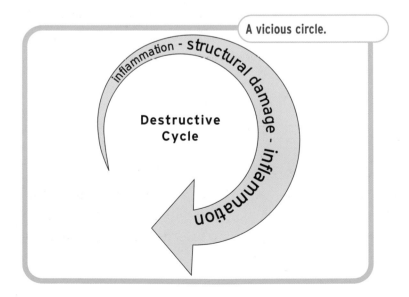

A vicious circle.

Inflammation - structural damage - inflammation

Destructive Cycle

# Can Cartilage Heal?

Cartilage has a limited blood supply and is under constant stress as your dog moves, so this tissue tends to not heal well. Most joints in the body normally are covered in **hyaline cartilage**. When cartilage is damaged, **fibrocartilage** often is formed in healing. The fibrocartilage is not as strong or as durable as hyaline cartilage. When there is severe cartilage damage (such as with hip dysplasia), cartilage very rarely heals. Many promising treatments are being developed to help cartilage healing, including the use of cartilage grafts and stem cells. Researchers hope to use these new treatments in the near future to manage osteoarthritis and other cartilage problems.

## Can We Stop the Progression of Osteoarthritis?

Successful treatment of your dog's osteoarthritis requires an end to the disease cycle. To do this, the cause of the disease must first be identified and treated, and the joint inflammation and deterioration stopped. The best chance of stopping osteoarthritis is when it is identified and treated early in the disease. Although the progression of osteoarthritis usually can't be stopped completely, with currently available treatments, the process can usually be slowed down quite a lot

# Osteoarthritis and Pain

Cartilage has no nerve endings. So why does osteoarthritis cause pain? Understanding the source of osteoarthritis pain will help you to make your dog more comfortable by helping you to understand how different treatments control pain.

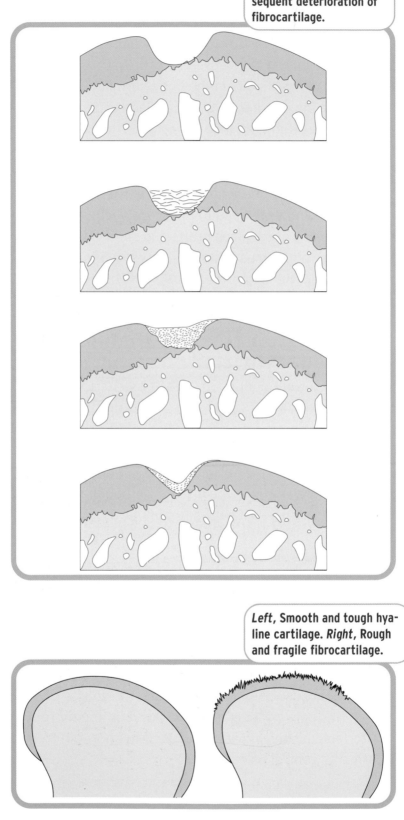

Cartilage healing and subsequent deterioration of fibrocartilage.

*Left*, Smooth and tough hyaline cartilage. *Right*, Rough and fragile fibrocartilage.

12

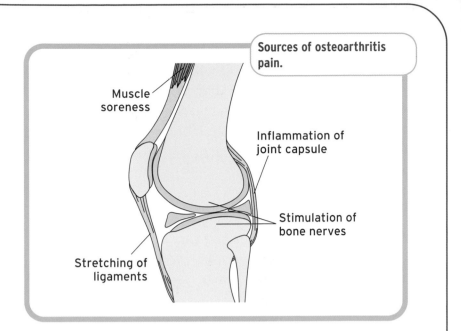

Sources of osteoarthritis pain.

Muscle soreness

Inflammation of joint capsule

Stimulation of bone nerves

Stretching of ligaments

Two major sources of pain are the nerves in the soft tissues surrounding the joint (the joint capsule) and the nerves in the bone underneath the cartilage (**subchondral bone**).

## Pain from the Joint Capsule

The joint capsule is a major source of pain in most dogs with osteoarthritis because it has many nerve endings on it and around it. Like any joint disease, osteoarthritis causes inflammation. This inflammation releases certain chemicals within the joint that stimulate nerve endings, causing pain. The degree of the inflammation

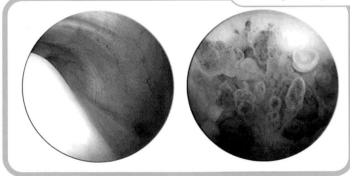

Arthroscopic view of a normal joint capsule *(left)* versus an inflamed joint capsule *(right)*.

and amount of pain depend on the type of disease and how severe it is. Joint infections and immune-mediated joint diseases (such as **lupus** or **rheumatoid arthritis**) can cause tremendous inflammation, with extreme pain. The inflammation of osteoarthritis is not usually as severe but can still be very painful.

Inflammation of the joint is not the only source of pain in osteoarthritis. Osteoarthritis leads to stiffening of the joint capsule **(fibrosis),** making it less flexible. This lack of flexibility means that your dog cannot move the joint as well or as fully as it should move. When a dog with osteoarthritis and thickened joint capsule tries to move the diseased joint normally, the joint capsule may stretch and tear, causing more pain.

### Pain from Bone

Pain from bone usually occurs in the later stages of osteoarthritis. There are sensitive nerve endings in the bone underneath the cartilage, but they usually are not stimulated until the cartilage disease is in a more severe stage. Think of bone pain in terms of teeth. Tooth enamel, like cartilage, has no nerve endings and is tough and durable. When the enamel layer of a tooth is injured, the tooth root is exposed. This makes it possible for the now-unprotected nerve endings in the root to be stimulated, causing serious pain. When the cartilage of a joint is damaged, exposing the bone underneath, then any stimulation of the nerve endings in the bone may cause serious pain, just as in the tooth. A lot of this stimulation or irritation in osteoarthritis comes from the inflammatory cells in the joint fluid. This fluid can reach your dog's bone nerves through cracks or holes in the cartilage after the

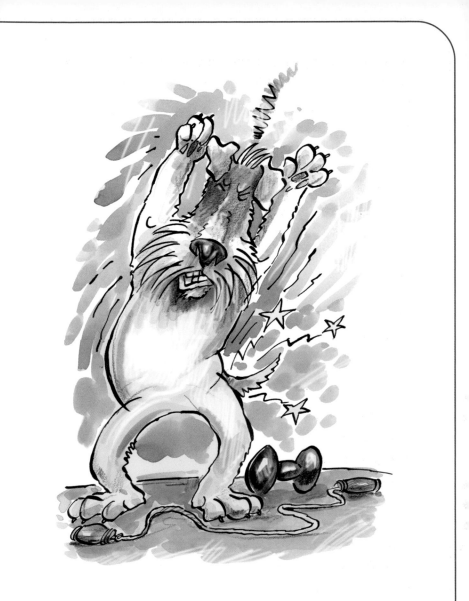

cartilage has worn away. In addition, once the cartilage is worn away on both surfaces of a joint, bone is then grinding on bone, causing even more stimulation of the bone's nerves. Increased blood flow within the bone next to the joint can also cause joint pain.

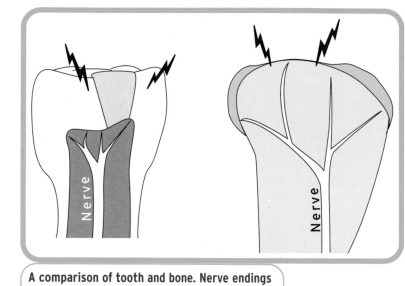

A comparison of tooth and bone. Nerve endings are stimulated below the bone when cartilage cover is lost or thin, causing pain.

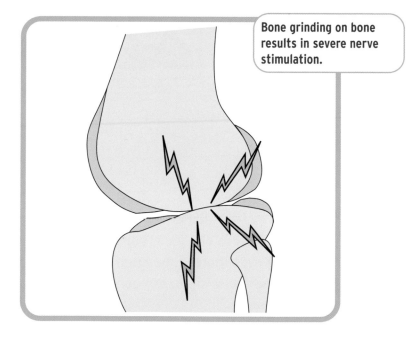

Bone grinding on bone results in severe nerve stimulation.

Now let's review the information in this chapter:

- **Osteoarthritis is also referred to as:**
  - **Arthritis**
  - **Osteoarthrosis**
  - **Degenerative joint disease, or DJD**
- **The cartilage matrix contains glucosamine and chondroitin, which you may have heard of as supplements for osteoarthritis. The matrix works as a shock absorber for the body.**
- **Osteoarthritis in dogs is usually caused by developmental diseases such as hip dysplasia.**
- **Cartilage does not heal easily.**
- **The pain of osteoarthritis comes from:**
  - **Stretching of the joint capsule**
  - **Nerve endings in the bone**
  - **Sore muscles**

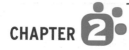

# SIGNS OF OSTEOARTHRITIS IN DOGS

We all understand that osteoarthritis causes pain and loss of function in ourselves and in our dogs. But in many cases osteoarthritis in a dog may not be recognized for months or even years. It is important to spot the signs of osteoarthritis as early as possible so that you and your veterinarian can decide which treatments will help give your dog a good quality of life for as long as possible. In this chapter we discuss the signs (your veterinarian may refer to these as the clinical signs) of osteoarthritis in dogs, paying special attention to signs that are often overlooked.

## Osteoarthritis and Pain

Osteoarthritis (OA) causes dogs to have pain and dysfunction in their joints. The first thing the pet owner should do is to control the pain, so it is important to know how to recognize it. The main signs of pain associated with osteoarthritis are:

- Lameness
- Difficulty rising

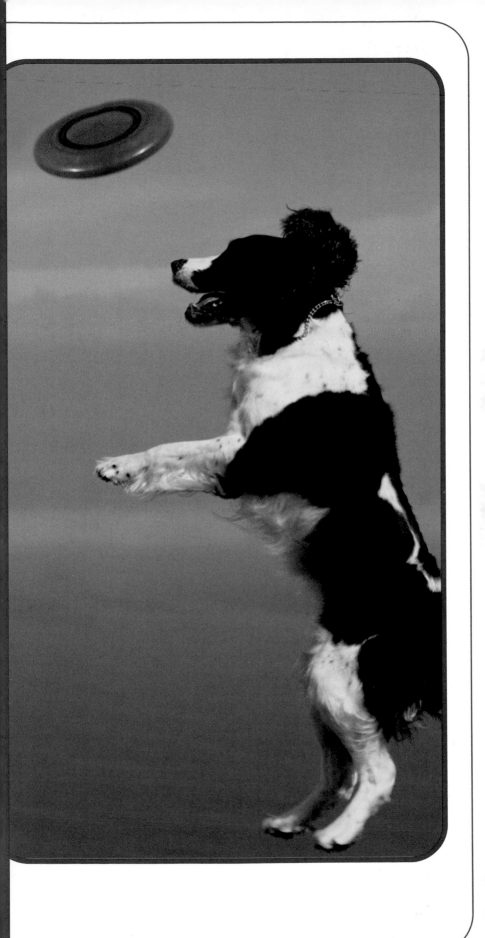

- Inability or unwillingness to exercise (exercise intolerance)
- Behavioral changes

# Lameness

**Lameness,** which is most often seen as a limp, is defined as the abnormal use of a limb. This means your dog is not using its legs properly. Lameness from osteoarthritis may be hard to see or may be very obvious. Some dog owners may think that although the lameness is obvious, their dog does not seem to be in any pain because they do not hear any whimpering or crying. Not true! Lameness is a response to pain and is an attempt by your pet to lessen her pain by changing the way she moves.

You can tell your dog has lameness in the forelimbs (front legs) by the "head nod." The head nod is a type of **gait abnormality**. In this gait abnormality, your dog lets her head drop down when the healthy limb strikes the ground and throws her head up when the sore limb strikes the ground. By doing this, your dog is trying to lessen the weight she places on her sore limb. Other forelimb gait abnormalities include taking longer or shorter steps and moving the limbs in an abnormal pattern (**circumduction**). With severe lameness, your dog may hold up the limb and avoid using it at all; however, lameness this bad is usually not associated with osteoarthritis.

Lameness of the hind limb may be more difficult to see. Gait abnormalities of the hind limb may include an increased vertical motion (called **hip hike**) and horizontal motion (**hip sway**) of the hips. Each of these "maneuvers" is an attempt by your dog to lessen the pain he feels

A head nod indicates a front leg lameness.

when walking by limiting the weight-bearing load and the motion of the arthritic joint. In the rear gait abnormality, your dog also will drop his head and extend his head forward in an attempt to shift weight to the forelimbs. Your dog may also shift weight off the affected leg when coming to a standstill. In other words, when coming to a stop, your dog will shift his weight to the opposite rear limb. You can tell your dog is weight shifting because the tarsal pad (the pad on your dog's ankle) will be lifted slightly off the ground when compared to the tarsal pad of the other rear limb. "**Bunny hopping,**" or use of both hind limbs together in a hopping manner, may be a sign that both hind limbs are affected (your dog is said to have **bilateral** involvement). Bunny hopping is usually associated with juvenile (puppy) hip dysplasia.

# Difficulty Rising

One of the most common signs of osteoarthritis is difficulty rising. Osteoarthritis causes stiffness of the joints through **fibrosis** or unusual thickening of the joint capsule. This makes the joints stiffer, making it harder for your dog to rise from a lying-down position.

Osteoarthritis can also lead to weakness in the muscles. Rising from a lying position requires a lot of muscu-

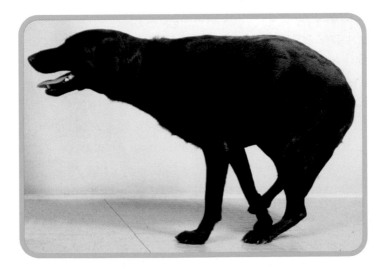

lar strength, so weakness of these muscles when your dog has osteoarthritis makes this movement slower and more difficult. Finally, rising puts a large weight load on the joints, worsening the pain of osteoarthritis. Difficulty rising happens most often when your dog has problems in one or both rear limbs or lower back. Dogs with these problems will usually pull themselves up with their forelimbs, rather than pushing up with their rear limbs.

Many dogs with osteoarthritis seem stiff when they first rise and begin moving but then appear to "warm up" and show fewer visible signs of pain. In these dogs, the symptoms come from the stiffness of the soft tissues (muscle and **ligaments**) around the joint and the large weight loads placed on the joints when they rise. When these dogs begin to move, however, their joints and muscles stretch and loosen, which relieves their discomfort and pain. Difficulty rising can happen with either hind limb osteoarthritis or forelimb osteoarthritis. Getting up from a resting position is even harder on slippery floors, so if your dog has difficulty rising, it is important to provide good footing to aid your dog. Dogs that repeatedly slip and fall may eventually become afraid of slippery surfaces such as tile or hardwood floors.

# Exercise Intolerance

Probably the most common but often overlooked sign of osteoarthritis is **exercise intolerance**. Many dogs with osteoarthritis may not show signs of lameness but will be unable or unwilling to exercise as long or hard as they have in the past. Many owners complain that their dog is reluctant to play with other dogs or to chase a ball or toy, as they had before. When walking, dogs with osteoarthritis will warm up and lose their stiffness but will eventually slow down—the owner may notice that the dog begins to lag behind on walks. On a long walk, the dog may try to turn around to go home or may simply lie down because of the pain of osteoarthritis. Owners may mistake this behavior as a sign of aging or poor conditioning; however, osteoarthritis should always be considered a possibility when a dog begins to exhibit a reluctance to exercise. Stair climbing also requires a lot of muscular strength and places large loads on the joints. A reluctance to climb stairs may be another sign of osteoarthritis.

With osteoarthritis, the muscles weaken and the soft tissues tighten, making exercise difficult and uncomfortable. In addition, although the pain of arthritis may at first decrease with warming up, it may later get worse after exercise because of the increased inflammation or swelling caused by joint movement.

# Behavioral Changes

Osteoarthritis can also appear as a change in your dog's behavior. Examples of behavior changes are aggressiveness toward family members or other pets and a desire to be left alone. The dog may wish to lie in an area of the house where it is quiet where there is little daily activity. A change in appetite might also be a sign that your dog is in discomfort or chronic pain.

# Osteoarthritis and Dysfunction

Dysfunction is the second major effect of osteoarthritis. When talking about osteoarthritis, **dysfunction** means the inability to move normally because of changes in the structures of the joints and limbs. Osteoarthritis can cause limb dysfunction in two important ways:

- **Decreased joint range of motion**
- **Muscular weakness**

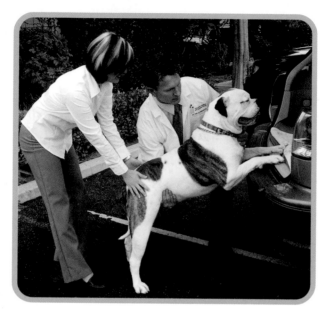

# Decreased Joint Range of Motion

As described before, osteoarthritis results in an increase in fibrous tissue in the joint capsule and surrounding structures (fibrosis). This fibrosis eventually leads to increased stiffness of the joint and a decrease in the **range of motion. Muscle atrophy** that comes from not using the muscle and tightness around the joint may also contribute to decreased range of motion. When this happens the dog cannot flex or extend the joint as much as normal. As a result, the dog may have a strange gait or method of sitting and may be unable to do previously normal activities such as jumping into a car and climbing stairs. A decreased range of motion also can be seen when examining your dog. It is easiest to recognize a decrease in range of motion when it is asymmetrical because you can use the opposite limb for comparison.

# Specific Changes in Range of Motion

When there is fibrosis around the joint, your dog will show fairly predictable changes in range of motion.

- **Shoulder–decrease in extension**
- **Elbow–decrease in flexion (ability to bend)**
- **Carpus (wrist)–decrease in flexion**
- **Hip–decrease in extension**
- **Knee–decrease in flexion**
- **Hock (ankle)-decrease in flexion**

The details of these changes are covered more completely in the chapters on the specific joints.

# Muscular Weakness

Muscular weakness associated with osteoarthritis represents a form of **disuse atrophy** (decrease in size due to lack of normal use). Because the dog is using the painful limb less, the muscles lose mass and then weaken. Generally there is no disease of the muscles themselves. This muscular weakness is exhibited by difficulty in rising and exercise intolerance.

The muscle wasting associated with osteoarthritis can almost always be reversed. Bringing the muscle back to its normal size and increasing flexibility and strength depends on the following factors:

- **Getting rid of or decreasing the pain of osteo-arthritis**
- **Restoring your dog's normal activity level**
- **Increasing your dog's range of motion**

You can tell your dog has muscle weakness when it has difficulty rising and exercising, and also by visually observ-

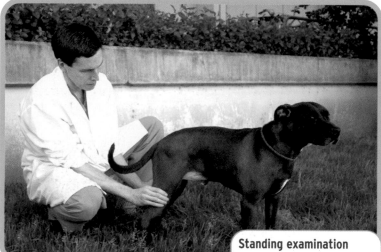

Standing examination in the dog.

## Assessment of Muscle Mass in Your Dog

Palpating or feeling for muscle mass on your dog is easiest to do with the dog standing. If possible, stand so that you can feel both sides at the same time. It is important that your dog stand as straight and symmetrically as possible so that the opposite legs are in similar positions.

Rub your hands over the shoulder regions to see if the bony bumps are more apparent on one side or the other. Do the same over the hip joints.

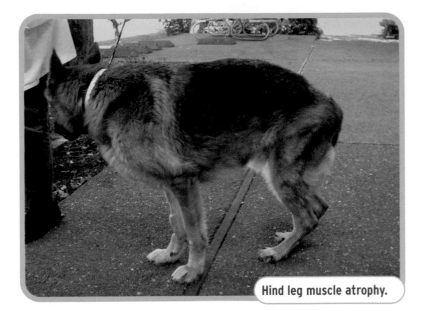

Hind leg muscle atrophy.

## Paradoxical Muscle Gain with Osteoarthritis

In addition to muscle loss, osteoarthritis can sometimes also lead to muscle gain. Dogs with severe and chronic osteoarthritis in the hind limbs often seem to have a very muscular chest and front limbs. This gain in muscle mass happens when the dog shifts its weight forward for easier walking.

ing decreased muscle size, or by feeling changes in the size of the muscles when **palpating** (or feeling) them (as described in the accompanying box). As with most changes, the visual and palpable changes can be seen best when they are unequal on both sides. The visual changes are also much easier to notice in short-haired dogs. Look carefully at the shoulder and hip regions, because changes in muscle mass in these locations are the easiest to recognize. Look for a bonier appearance that can mean there has been a loss of muscle mass.

Loss of muscle mass can be felt most easily in the shoulder and hip regions. Remember that osteoarthritis anywhere in a limb will cause loss of muscle mass in the *entire* limb and not just around the affected joint. So loss of muscle around the shoulder, for example, does not necessarily mean your dog has shoulder arthritis; the muscle loss may instead be a result of osteoarthritis of the elbow or **carpus** (wrist). By the same token, muscle loss around the hip does not necessarily mean your dog has osteoarthritis of the hip, but may be caused by problems of the knee or **hock** (ankle). Also keep in mind that muscle loss may be caused by other orthopedic, neurologic, or metabolic diseases.

Watching changes in muscle mass is a painless and excellent way to determine how effective therapy is. When

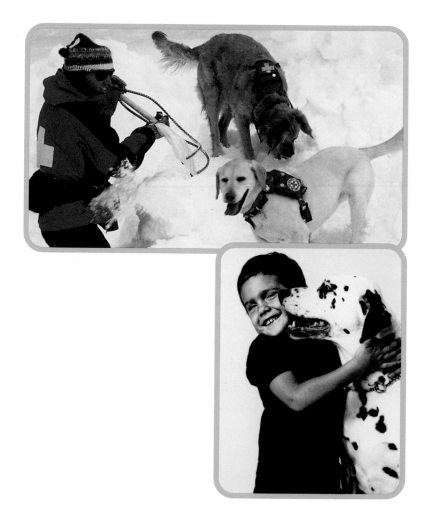

your dog's osteoarthritis therapy is effective, you should notice gradual improvement in exercise level, less effort in rising, and increased muscle mass.

# Variations in Response

One of the hardest things about managing osteoarthritis is that each individual dog responds to the disease differently. Just as with people, some dogs are extremely sensitive to the pain of osteoarthritis, and some are extremely brave and show no signs of pain. As an excellent example, a study of dogs used in the military showed that even though they had severe osteoarthritis, most dogs were willing and able to perform their working duties. On the other hand, certain dogs exhibit extreme lameness and exercise intolerance even with relatively mild degrees of osteoarthritis.

# Quality of Life

**Quality of life** when talking about osteoarthritis means the minimization of pain. The goal of management of your dog's osteoarthritis is to get rid of or minimize the pain your dog feels during normal daily activities. In some cases, you can control your dog's pain by decreasing the amount of force felt on the joints (through weight reduction and exercise moderation), increasing joint range of motion (with physical therapy), and medication (medication may not be the first option you'll want to consider). However, in other cases, your dog's pain may be so bad that it requires surgery. You, as the owner, with your veterinarian's help, must decide when your dog's pain and discomfort are worth the cost and risks of these treatments.

## Where We Stand

The goal of osteoarthritis management is based on two concerns: quality of life and function. Dog owners are in the best position to judge their dog's quality of life, and they are the ones who know how well their pet is functioning.

Although your veterinarian can help you in recognizing pain in your dog and in deciding on the best therapy, you are the best judge and must make the final decisions about the management of this disease and its effects on your dog.

# Function

"Adequate" function means different things to different people. For many pet owners, their dog is primarily a companion, but other dogs have roles in hunting, agility competitions, or activities such as search and rescue. Age also factors into what is considered adequate function. Most dog owners do not expect the same function from a 14-year-old dog as they do from a 2-year-old.

Although naturally the veterinarian will want to restore full activity to every dog, owners should clearly explain their expectations for what they consider adequate function of their dog.

Now let's review the information in this chapter:

- **The most common signs of osteoarthritis are:**
  - **Lameness, or limping**
  - **Difficulty getting up**
  - **Not wanting to exercise as much as before**
  - **Changes in behavior**
- **In a dog with a lame front leg, the head goes up when the painful limb hits the ground.**
- **A dog that "bunny hops" may have sore hind legs.**
- **Difficulty getting up is a common sign of osteoarthritis.**
- **Not wanting to exercise is probably the most overlooked sign of osteoarthritis.**
- **A dog with osteoarthritis is often less flexible in the arthritic joint, and the muscles in that leg may be weak.**
- **For the owner of a dog with osteoarthritis, the two most important things to consider are the dog's quality of life and the dog's ability to function in daily life.**

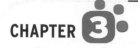

# GENERAL CAUSES OF OSTEOARTHRITIS IN DOGS

In this chapter we review the common causes of osteoarthritis and talk about how some of them can be prevented. Osteoarthritis is caused when disease or injury affects your dog's joint or joints. In dogs, osteoarthritis is usually caused by inherited diseases of development such as hip or elbow dysplasia. A ruptured cruciate ligament in the knee is another common cause of osteoarthritis in dogs. It's important to understand the causes of osteoarthritis because getting rid of the cause is a critical step in keeping arthritis from getting worse.

The specific cause of a dog's osteoarthritis is considered either **developmental** or **acquired.** Developmental causes are those that are due to poor genes (genetics) or birth defects, and acquired causes are those that are due to injury or diseases such as infection or cancer.

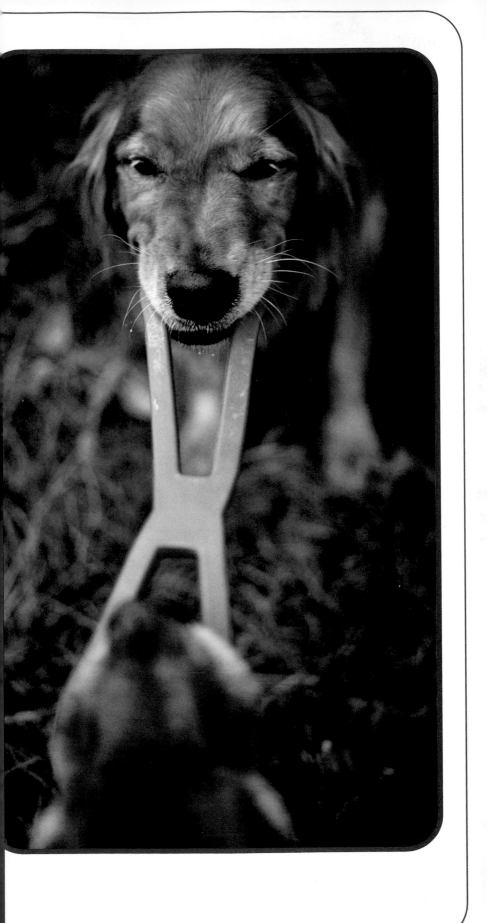

| Congenital/Developmental versus Acquired Causes of Osteoarthritis | |
|---|---|
| **Congenital/ Developmental** | **Acquired** |
| Dysplasia<br>Congenital defects | Trauma<br>Infections<br>Immune-mediated joint disorders<br>Cancer |

# Congenital and Developmental Conditions Associated with Osteoarthritis

Osteoarthritis that is caused by disorders that affect the growth or structure of joints is either congenital or developmental. Congenital disorders are present in a dog at birth. Developmental disorders occur as a dog's skeleton grows. Examples of developmental disorders are:

- **Hip dysplasia**
- **Elbow dysplasia**
- **Osteochondritis dissecans**

It is also possible that **cranial cruciate ligament** rupture may be a developmental disease, but this is still widely debated.

## What Is Dysplasia?

**Dysplasia** means "abnormal development." The most common dysplasias in dogs are hip dysplasia and elbow dysplasia. In both cases, a malformation in the joint devel-

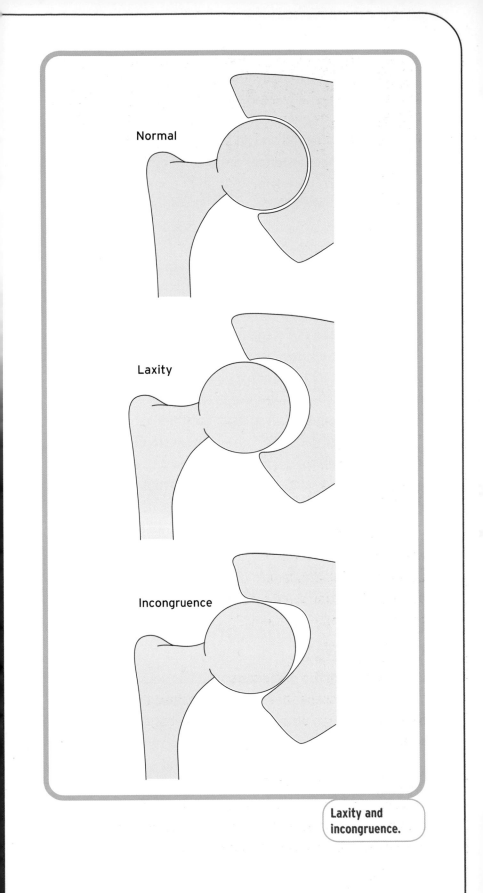

Normal

Laxity

Incongruence

Laxity and
incongruence.

ops as the dog's skeleton grows. This malformation may be mild or severe. If your dog has only mild dysplasia, you may never notice any signs of pain or discomfort.

In dysplasia, the type of joint malformation depends on which joint is affected. In the elbow joint, the type of malformation is **incongruence**, or poor fit, but in the hip joint, the malformation is a combination of poor fit <u>and</u> joint **laxity**, or looseness. Think of a metal door hinge. A well-made hinge will work for many years without a problem, whereas a poorly made hinge will sag and its moving parts will begin to show signs of wear. The cartilage in a poorly developed joint will begin to wear prematurely for the same reason. The basic causes of canine hip and elbow dysplasia are still not clear, but abnormalities of a dog's genes (genetic causes) are the most likely cause. External environmental factors such as being overweight or inappropriate exercise or a lack of exercise can definitely contribute to the signs of dysplasia, but they cannot cause dysplasia. Dysplasia is definitely a **genetic disease.**

The treatment of dysplasia depends on how bad the dysplasia is and on the affected joint. Treatment can be both medical and surgical. Prevention is very difficult and requires being able to identify which dogs are likely to pass on poor genes. Improving environmental factors like weight and activity level may help lessen the signs of dysplastic diseases, but they will not eliminate it.

# What Is Osteochondritis Dissecans?

**Osteochondritis dissecans** (OCD) is caused by a problem in cartilage as it develops. Other species besides dogs can have OCD, and the cause varies depending on the species. For instance, in humans, OCD often occurs in children who are involved in gymnastics and baseball pitching (ever heard of "Little League elbow"?). It is caused by the activity's trauma on young, growing cartilage. In pigs, OCD is caused by overfeeding and fast growth. In dogs, the causes seem to be genetics and nutrition.

In growing dogs, much of the bones are actually made up of cartilage. As the dog becomes full-grown, most of the cartilage changes to true bone, except for the thin layer of cartilage at the ends of the bone (joint surfaces). This tissue lets joints move and glide smoothly, without much friction. In OCD, part of this cartilage remains thickened. Both genetics and nutrition seem to cause this problem. Genetically, certain breeds such as Labrador Retrievers and Golden Retrievers are more likely to develop OCD. Nutritionally, feeding too many calories and too much calcium contributes to OCD in dogs. The zone of thickened cartilage is easily injured because this area is not well joined with the bone underneath. Even normal activities such as running can cause the cartilage to separate from the underlying bone. This causes a cartilage flap to form—an area of cartilage that is attached to the underlying bone in some places but torn in others. **Joint fluid** seeps underneath the cartilage and irritates nerve endings in the underlying bone, causing pain. The separated section of cartilage rubs against the cartilage surface opposite it, causing osteoarthritis to develop. As long as the separated cartilage is there, healing is not possible.

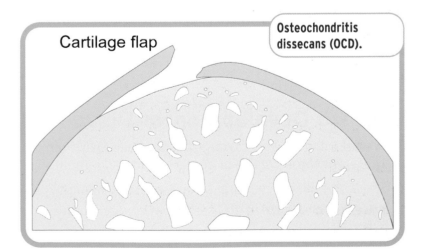

Cartilage flap

Osteochondritis dissecans (OCD).

## Where We Stand

Current evidence strongly shows that genetics are the major cause of dysplasias and osteochondritis dissecans (OCD). These diseases may be worsened by fast growth as a result of feeding too many calories and by improper exercise—but these factors cannot *cause* joint dysplasia or OCD.

We strongly encourage dog owners to let the breeder know whenever a purebred dog has a developmental disease, because breeders have a responsibility to breed to eliminate these diseases.

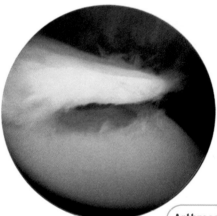

Arthroscopic view of a shoulder joint with a cartilage flap.

## How Do Developmental Diseases Begin?

There are three causes of congenital/developmental diseases in dogs:

- Genetics
- Nutrition
- Environmental factors

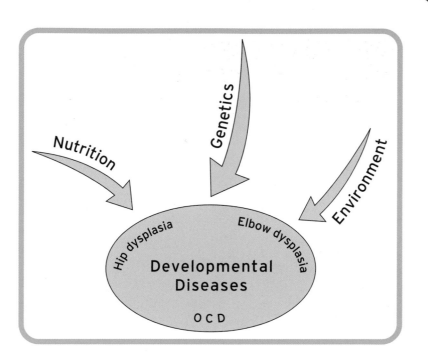

## Genetics

Poor genetics is the most common cause of developmental joint diseases in dogs. The specific joint problem is not always clear, but genetic flaws do seem to lead to joint problems, from subtle to severe. The joints become damaged as they are used, resulting in osteoarthritis.

It is difficult to spot the genetic problems that cause osteoarthritis. Because of this, it is hard to say which dogs should and should not be bred in order to eliminate these diseases. Veterinary organizations have worked for many years to outline ways of identifying dogs that carry genes connected to joint disease, and to help dog breeders to rid their lines of these genes. These organizations are discussed in the accompanying section "How to Find an Orthopedically Healthy Puppy: Guidelines for Success."

## Nutrition

Improper nutrition has been shown to increase the severity of diseases such as hip dysplasia and OCD. Improper nutrition alone cannot cause these conditions—but nutrition-related problems may make the disease worse.

# Diet, Osteoarthritis, and Longevity

   Recently veterinarians from the University of Pennsylvania, Cornell University, and England, working with Nestle-Purina, reported their results from a study of the effects of diet on hip dysplasia and length of life. The researchers separated a group of 48 Labrador Retrievers into two groups. In the first group, the dogs were allowed to eat as much as they wanted. Dogs in the second group were allowed to eat only 75% as much as the first group. This intensive study followed all the dogs for their entire lives. In the end, the dogs that ate less had a great deal less osteoarthritis of the hips than the dogs that ate more. Also, the dogs that ate less lived much longer. These results prove that healthy body weight allows dogs to live longer and healthier lives with less chance of osteoarthritis.

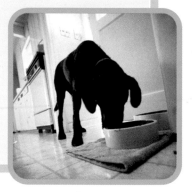

The most common nutrition errors dog owners make are feeding too many calories and incorrectly supplementing their dog's diet. In puppies, feeding too many calories and supplementing the diet improperly contribute to too-fast growth. Rapid growth of a puppy's skeleton with poor muscular and soft tissue development puts extra strain on the bones and joints. This extra strain aggravates joint disease and dysplasia. In adult dogs, extra body weight makes the signs of osteoarthritis much worse and may speed the disease's progress.

### Environmental Factors

Environmental factors don't often contribute to genetic and developmental joint diseases, and it is very important that dog owners not blame themselves for these diseases.

The only environmental factor that noticeably affects osteoarthritis is the amount and type of exercise. It is impossible for exercise to cause diseases such as hip dysplasia, elbow dysplasia, or OCD. But improper exercise can worsen the signs and even speed up the disease process. If you suspect your puppy has a joint disease, limit its activity to leash walking until your veterinarian can examine and evaluate your puppy.

A proper exercise routine, home physical therapy, and professional physical therapy are excellent tools for managing your dog's osteoarthritis. However, the timing and use of these treatments depend on the status and the

Extra body weight is the number one preventable factor of osteoarthritic pain, discomfort, and loss of function.

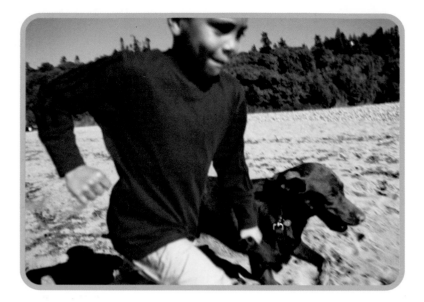

stage of the disease in each individual joint. Generally, you should restrict your dog's activity to leash walking and discourage rough playing and jumping until your veterinarian has diagnosed your dog and developed a treatment plan.

# Acquired Causes of Osteoarthritis

There are four acquired causes of osteoarthritis:

- **Traumatic injuries**
- **Infection**
- **Immune-mediated joint disease**
- **Cancer**

## Trauma

Injury is the most common cause of acquired joint disease. Traumatic injuries that can lead to joint osteoarthritis are:

- **Vehicle accidents (such as being hit by a car)**
- **Falls**
- **Bite wounds**

Osteoarthritis can be caused by injuries that change the formation of a normal joint. These types of injuries include:

- **Fractures**
- **Ligament damage**
- **Joint dislocation**
- **Direct cartilage damage**

In most cases, trauma is obvious because these injuries are very painful. If you suspect your pet has been injured in some way, contact your veterinarian as quickly as possible. Joint trauma often needs

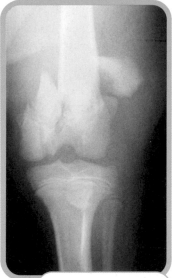

X-ray of a fractured joint.

immediate medical attention, with surgical repair performed as soon as your pet's condition is stable.

## Fractures

Joint fractures cause damage to the joint surface and cartilage. They almost always require surgery. Surgical correction is usually needed right away for your dog to heal properly. If the joint surfaces remain out of align-

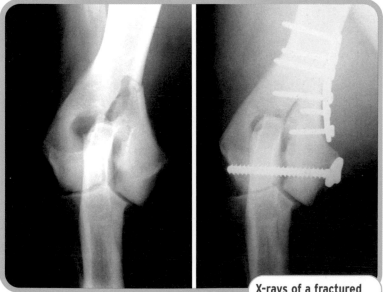

X-rays of a fractured joint before and after surgical repair.

ment for too long, the affected cartilage and bone will be damaged forever, leading to severe osteoarthritis. On the other hand, if joint fractures are successfully repaired with surgery, minimal osteoarthritis will result in most cases.

### Ligament Damage

Joints are held in position by the ligaments that surround them. Ligaments are commonly damaged when joints are injured—for example, the **collateral ligaments** of the ankle or knee. The most common ligament injury for dogs is the stretching or tearing of the **cranial cruciate ligament** (CCL) of the knee. In humans, this same ligament is called the anterior cruciate ligament (ACL).

Just as in humans, ligament damage causes sudden pain in dogs. The pain is a result of the ligament tearing and of the surrounding soft tissues stretching. Without the healthy ligament, the joint becomes unstable. Soft tissues around the joint, such as the joint capsule, and other ligaments, nerves, and blood vessels are stretched, caus-

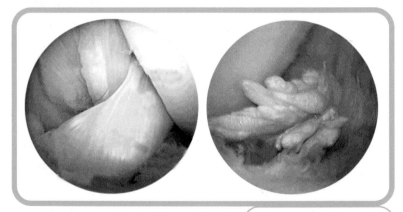

Arthroscopic views of a normal cruciate ligament *(left)* and a torn ligament *(right).*

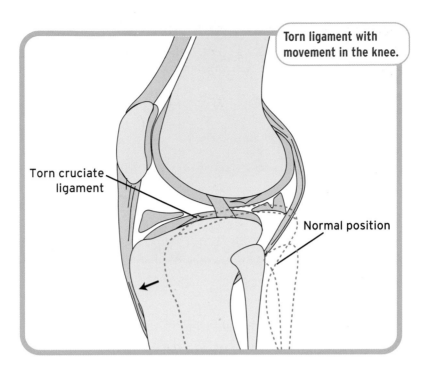

**Torn ligament with movement in the knee.**

Torn cruciate ligament

Normal position

ing pain. The pain can be relieved temporarily by stabilizing the joint with a bandage, or permanently with surgery.

When ligament injury has made a joint unstable, the joint surfaces rub against each other improperly. This motion causes cartilage damage and leads to the onset of osteoarthritis. Immediate repair of joint instability is key to maintaining a healthy joint, because the course of osteoarthritis is difficult to stop, and damaged cartilage cannot heal well.

## Joint Luxation

**Luxation** (dislocation) of a joint occurs frequently in dogs; the most commonly affected joints are the hip and the elbow. The initial pain is severe and is a result of stretching and tearing the surrounding soft tissue, as with other ligament trauma. Joint luxation is different from ligament damage like a CCL injury. In dislocations, the bones that make up the joint must be moved back into their normal position. This procedure is called **reduction**.

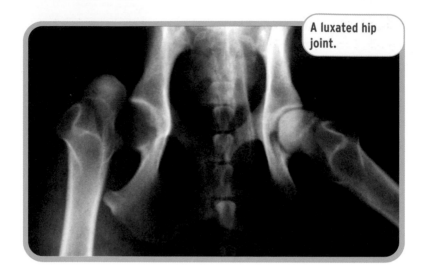

A luxated hip joint.

If the dislocation is not treated, the joint surfaces wear down as the joint moves. Surface cartilage is damaged as a result. To prevent this, the dislocation needs to be repaired, or reduced, and the joint must be stabilized as soon as possible. Reduction requires general anesthesia, and surgery may be needed to keep the joint in normal position. With certain joints, dislocation often needs surgery—for example, the shoulder, wrist, knee, and ankle. Dislocation of other joints, such as the hip and the elbow, may be managed without surgery. But if non-surgical treatment does not work, surgery will be needed.

## Infection

Infection of a joint does not happen often in dogs. Injuries that penetrate the joint, such as bite wounds and previous surgery, are possible causes of joint infection. A very ill dog's joint can suddenly become infected without a penetrating injury, but this is rare.

Joint infection needs immediate treatment. Antibiotics are used to treat mild infections. Surgery is needed to treat more severe infections. Bacteria can quickly destroy joint cartilage, so it is extremely important to remove bacteria from the joint as quickly as possible. Late treatment or poor treatment will lead to breakdown of the cartilage and severe osteoarthritis. Treatment of severe joint infection involves antibiotics and draining the infected fluid from the joint and rinsing the joint space thoroughly with sterile fluid. The choice of antibiotic may be based on culture and sensitivity studies, where the bacteria attacking the joint are grown in the lab in order to see what antibiotic will effectively destroy them.

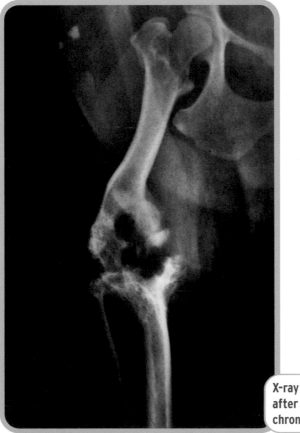

X-ray of a joint after severe chronic infection.

# Immune-Mediated Joint Disease

Immune-mediated joint disease in dogs is similar to the same disease in humans. Systemic lupus erythematosus (lupus) and rheumatoid arthritis are examples of immune-mediated joint diseases. In **lupus** and **rheumatoid arthritis,** the body produces cells that attack the cartilage surface. We do not know the reason for this abnormal immune response, but it may be a result of infection, digestive system disease, or cancer. Sometimes there is no other additional disease.

Immune-mediated joint disease is painful and may affect any breed of dog, and there are breed-specific forms of immune-mediated conditions. Small dogs get the disease in multiple joints, including the wrist and ankle. Immune-mediated joint disease is diagnosed using an analysis of joint fluid, x-ray studies, and assessment of the dog's physical condition and behavior. Once the disease is diagnosed, it is important to look for any related diseases, but the underlying cause of the joint disease often is not identified.

Because the immune-mediated joint disease destroys cartilage, osteoarthritis begins to develop. Therefore, this disease should be controlled as quickly as possible. Treatment may be medical (non-surgical) in mild to moderate cases but may involve surgery in more severe cases. **Steroids** or stronger medications are used to control the body's immune system in medical treatment. Preventing the cartilage-attacking cells from developing will stop the joint swelling and destruction. Once the disease is under control, frequent rechecks and monitoring are needed to ensure that long-term treatment is working. If treatment is late or poor, the destruction of joint cartilage will cause significant joint pain. If this occurs, surgery (**arthrodesis** or fusion) is needed to repair the joint.

# Cancer

Rarely, osteoarthritis and joint pain can be the first signs of cancer. Cancer of the surrounding bone and cancer of the joint capsule are the most common types. Joint cancer is rare, so owners should not be too worried about this possibility.

Now let's review the information in this chapter:

- **In most dogs, osteoarthritis results from developmental causes—problems in joint development while the dog is growing. This kind of genetic abnormality is often called dysplasia (hip dysplasia, elbow dysplasia), which means "abnormal development."**
- **Another common cause of osteoarthritis in dogs is rupture of the cruciate ligament of the knee. It's not known what causes this injury.**
- **Trauma, infection, and immune diseases also cause osteoarthritis in dogs.**
- **Before shopping for a purebred puppy, learn about the diseases that affect the breed you want and find a reputable breeder.**

# Getting a Healthy Puppy or Dog

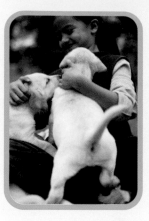

When a person thinks about getting a puppy, joint disease usually isn't a main concern. However, understanding some basic facts about breeding and joint disease can save money and prevent heartache down the road. Many future dog owners may choose to adopt dogs from humane shelters, where the background of the dog is unknown, while other people look for purebred dogs from a pet store or breeder. When possible, it pays to do your homework and follow the steps outlined in the following section, "How to Find an Orthopedically Healthy Puppy: Guidelines for Success" to reduce the risk of joint disease for your new dog.

## How to Find an Orthopedically Healthy Puppy
### Guidelines for Success
#### AUTUMN P. DAVIDSON

Once you have decided to get a purebred dog, the challenging search for that puppy begins. These guidelines are meant to help you become an informed puppy shopper. An informed puppy shopper knows about the genetic problems common in the breed he or she wants to buy. An informed puppy shopper also is familiar with the ways breeders try to prevent breeding dogs with those problems. Good breeders and informed puppy shoppers are both very concerned about genetic joint problems, such as 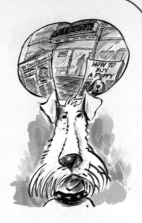 hip and elbow dysplasia. Last, an informed puppy shopper knows what to look for in terms of a puppy's general health, personality, and socialization, or how comfortable the puppy is with new people, animals, and situations.

The best purebred puppies usually are bought from a reputable breeder. Finding a reputable breeder with puppies available can be challenging. Finding a reputable breeder of purebred dogs is the most important first step toward buying a healthy and high-quality puppy.

## Where Can Purebred Dogs Be Found?

Actually, a purebred dog usually can be found quite easily. The classified sections of most newspapers often have many advertisements for purebred puppies, usually at reasonable prices. Some pet shops sell purebred puppies, usually at higher prices. The Internet is another way to find available purebred puppies. Roadside signs steer unprepared puppy shoppers to backyard litters. Offering puppies for sale at flea markets and parking lots takes advantage of the compassion of impulse buyers.

Although a puppy from one of these sources can be wonderful, the chances of getting a healthy, good-quality puppy are much higher if the puppy is bought from a reputable breeder, using appropriate networking.

Reputable breeders do not need to advertise in the newspaper and consider it unethical to sell puppies through pet shops. They may post information about their kennel on the Internet but would never sell a puppy through the Internet without a personal interview with the potential buyer. Reputable breeders depend on "word of mouth" advertising, generally through a referral network of breeders ("Sorry, I do not have any yellow Labrador Retriever puppies available, but I can refer you to another reputable breeder") and from veterinary and other dog professionals who know them personally.

## What Is a Reputable Breeder?

A reputable breeder tries very hard to produce the best-quality puppies possible. Quality in this sense means that the puppies are in good health, have few genetic defects and good temperaments, and display their breed's known and desired traits.

Most reputable breeders breed dogs as a hobby. They spend time at competitive dog events, either against other dogs or their owners or against a performance standard. They breed dogs to produce winners or successful workers for competitions. Because dogs tend to have litters rather than single puppies, "extra" puppies result when breeders mate two dogs to produce what they hope will be a winner or a successful worker. As a result, puppies are available for the public. What makes breeders reputable is what they do professionally that shows compassion for their breed. Reputable breeders want to produce wonderful dogs, not only for their own use but for the public as well. They work hard to overcome the unavoidable genetic flaws of the purebred dog. Reputable breeders also do not want to contribute to the dog overpopulation problem by producing extra puppies, and would be devastated to learn that one of their puppies ended up in a shelter or as a stray.

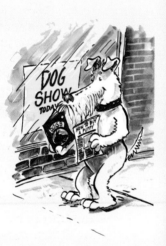

Breeders who produce puppies purely for financial gain or personal glory may be so determined to win competi-

# Characteristics of Reputable Breeders

- Are completely knowledgeable about their breed (appearance, disposition, genetics, breed-specific traits, history)
- Are willing to give you references (veterinarians, previous puppy buyers, other breeders)
- Interview hopeful puppy buyers carefully
- Are more interested in the quality of the home you can offer than in the puppy's sale price
- Will refuse to sell a puppy to an unfit home or to breed a dog that should not reproduce
- Breed to improve their line of dogs
- Are always willing to take back a puppy/dog that does not work out with a purchaser
- Are knowledgeable about puppy training, puppy medical problems, and good local veterinarians and kennels
- Know their dogs' family background; provide accurate pedigrees, appropriate registration papers, and medical and genetic records on puppies
- Follow up on puppy placements and are available to you for questions and concerns after the purchase is complete—even years later
- Collect and keep accurate health and temperament (personality) records about the long-term outcome of their breedings
- Help fight the canine overpopulation problem by supporting rescue groups for the breed
- Participate in the dog fancy world somehow, as it is their hobby
- Prove the quality of the dogs they've bred, through titles, certificates, and health evaluations
- Encourage or require neutering of puppies they sell
- Take excellent care of their dogs in terms of housing, husbandry, health care, and loving interaction
- Are financially able and willing to support their dog breeding hobby
- Have firm knowledge about individual puppies in a litter and help the puppy shopper to pick the puppy that is the best match, rather than simply letting the shopper pick a puppy impulsively
- Usually have more hopeful puppy buyers than puppies available, resulting in waiting lists; the prices of their puppies reflect their quality
- Are ethical

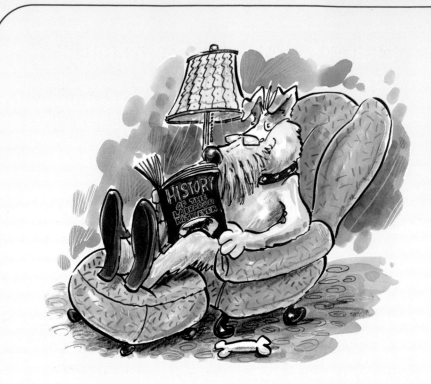

tions that they are not concerned about extra, lower-quality puppies produced while they pursue that hobby. "Puppy mills" are the worst of breeders. Their goal is mass puppy production, and they will market their "product" however is easiest (pet shops, Internet, magazines).

"Backyard" breeders breed pets and are not involved in competitive dog events. Backyard breeders can be either reputable or disreputable. Some backyard breeders breed their pet because they believe that it is a wonderful example of the breed and should be bred to produce more. They may or may not have done homework to judge the dog's genetic health and whether it is a truly desirable breed representative.

## What Should an Informed Puppy Shopper Know about Genetic Orthopedic Problems?

Reputable breeders screen dogs for genetic joint problems that are common to the breed and use only healthy dogs for breeding. Testing for orthopedic disease typically involves taking x-ray films of hips and elbows and sometimes shoulders and hocks. General veterinarians often evaluate the x-ray films first, but most breeders send the x-ray films to a central registry so that they may be compared and measured against an established standard for their breed. These registries include the Orthopedic Foundation for Animals (OFA), the University of Pennsylvania Hip Improvement Program (PennHIP), and the Institute for Genetic Disease Control. Registries provide consistent methods to judge x-ray films and are a reliable source for the public to research dogs used for breeding. Breeders participating in such registries have reduced genetic orthopedic diseases, which means that they are breeding only dogs that are genetically normal. Many pure-breed dog clubs have a code of ethics that includes guidelines for breeding. These guidelines usually require that dogs used for breeding have x-ray studies performed to screen for common genetic orthopedic diseases once they're fully grown, and that the x-ray results be normal. Unfortunately, hip dysplasia and elbow dysplasia are still very common because some breeders believe that looking at the hips of a dog's parents, grandparents, and great-grandparents will lead to improvements in the breed, when in fact a professional should judge the hips of the dog's siblings and half-siblings.

## Registry Resources

Orthopedic Foundation for Animals (OFA)
2300 E. Nifong Boulevard
Columbia, MO 65201-3856
*Phone*: (573) 442-0418
*Fax*: (573) 875-5073
*E-mail*: ofa@offa.org
*Web site*: www.offa.org

PennHIP (University of Pennsylvania Hip
Improvement Program)
Administrative Center
3900 Delancy Street
Philadelphia, PA 19104
*Phone*: (215) 573-3176
*E-mail*: pennhipinfo@pennhip.org
*Web site*: www.pennhip.org

It is important for puppy shoppers to understand the difference between phenotype and genotype. The dog's physical features and overall physical condition make up that dog's phenotype. For example, hips that are phenotypically normal have a femur (thigh bone) that fits normally into the hip socket, with no signs of arthritis or laxity (looseness). A dog's genotype, on the other hand, is the genetic makeup of that dog. It is possible for dogs with phenotypically normal hips to have some genes for hip dysplasia. This is why seemingly normal dogs, with a normal pheno-

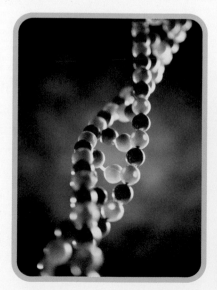

## Phenotype versus Genotype

The phenotype is the dog's set of actual physical traits. Genotype is the genetic code that decides the physical traits.

type according to a hip x-ray film, can still produce puppies that develop dysplasia.

Private breeders tend to decide which dogs to breed according to their appearance, genetic health, and ability to perform (the order of importance varies with the breeder). Fewer genetic problems occur when dogs used for breeding come from litters with normal genes in all of the littermates, rather than from dogs whose parents and grandparents were normal, but whose littermates were abnormal or whose status was unknown. In fact, puppies are likely to be genetically healthy only if breeding dogs are chosen from litters in which all the littermates are phenotypically normal. The phenotypes of a dog's littermates tell more about that dog's genotype than the status of its parents. Unfortunately, as long as breeders select dogs for breeding according to their individual phenotype, physical appearance, and performance, instead of the littermates' genetic health, genetic orthopedic disorders will continue to be a big problem.

In summary, the likelihood of a specific dog's producing puppies with joint problems should be judged by evaluating the littermates, not the great-grandparents, grandparents, and parents. Dysplasia is much less common among dogs born to parents that have genetically healthy littermates. Because of this, it is important for informed puppy shoppers to ask about the siblings of the parents of the litter, as well as asking for paperwork proving the absence of a specific genetic disorder for the parents. By asking the proper questions, the puppy shopper will encourage more accurate genetic screening by breeders.

## What Resources Are Available to an Informed Puppy Shopper?

Prospective puppy shoppers should learn all about the breed they wish to buy before visiting breeders. Veterinarians and animal behaviorists can provide basic information about the health and personality characteristics of a breed. The American Kennel Club (AKC), the largest registry of purebred dogs in the United States, has information on specific-breed health issues through the Canine Health Information Center (CHIC), at www.caninehealthinfo.org.

Keep in mind: This information is limited to only the defects that the AKC considers "heritable and significant" for the breed and may not cover everything. The CHIC provides lists of dogs that have "earned" a CHIC number by passing the AKC breed requirements, along with evaluations available for close relatives. This provides important information about the dog's genetically healthy relatives but nothing about the relatives that were not found to be normal or that were not evaluated at all. The informed puppy shopper should recognize that this information is incomplete in judging a litter's genetic health.

The OFA (www.ofa.org) and the Canine Eye Registry Foundation (www.vetpurdue.edu~yshen/cerf.html) also have Web sites providing information about dogs that have been evaluated and registered as normal. They also provide statistics for particular genetic diseases based on their data. Unfortunately, data on affected dogs can be made public only if the breeder allows it. As a result, genetic diseases are underreported.

The PennHIP registry has an informative Web site, where puppy shoppers can learn about this registry's method of evaluating dogs for hip dysplasia, at www.pennhip.org.

National and local breed clubs are available on the Internet as well and offer good breed-specific information for puppy shoppers.

Finally, you can obtain the most current information about breed-specific genetic disease from academic veterinarians (usually associated with veterinary schools) who are researching the disorders.

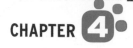

# GENERAL DIAGNOSIS OF OSTEOARTHRITIS

**Your veterinarian can often diagnose osteoarthritis just by hearing your description of your dog's pain and disability. In other cases, though, the diagnosis is much more challenging. Your veterinarian has many tools to investigate your dog's joints—radiography, fluid analysis, arthroscopy, MRI, CT—but the hands are a veterinarian's most important tool in evaluating a dog's joints. An experienced veterinarian can detect changes in the muscles, ligaments, and joints that will point to a diagnosis. In this chapter we take a look at the methods used to diagnose osteoarthritis in dogs.**

# Patient History

The owner of a dog with osteoarthritis usually tells the veterinarian that the animal is lame or limping, does not seem to want to exercise as much as she has in the past, and has difficulty getting up. A dog with osteoarthritis may be stiffest on getting up after sleeping, although the dog's stiffness often gets better after a few minutes of gentle movement. A dog with osteoarthritis may also seem to have mild to severe **lameness** after lots of exercise. The dog may have had an injury earlier in life or may have had orthopedic surgery in the past, or **dysplasia** may have been diagnosed earlier in life.

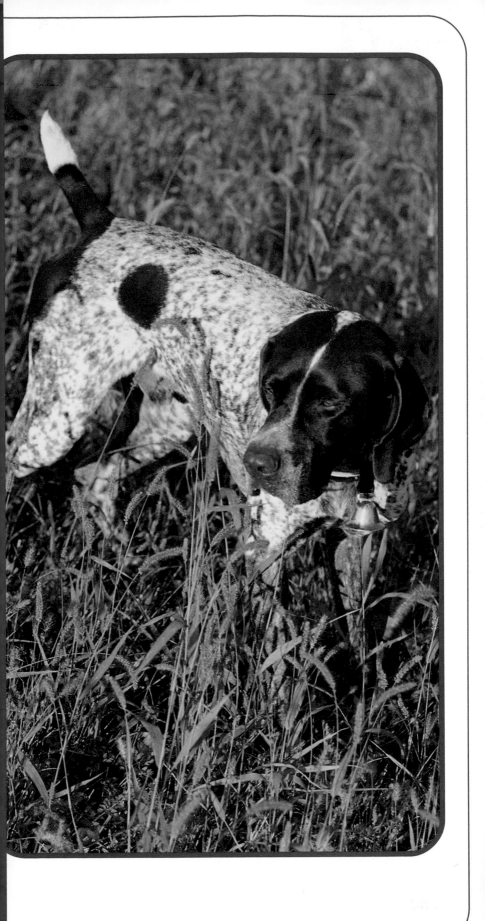

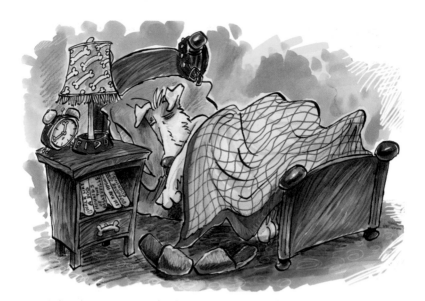

# Patient Examination

Both a general physical examination and an orthopedic examination are important in the diagnosis and treatment of osteoarthritis. A thorough general examination will help make sure that you and your dog's veterinarian are aware of all of the dog's problems, which will help you make the best decisions about the treatment of osteoarthritis and any other diseases or disorders your veterinarian may find.

The orthopedic examination usually starts with your veterinarian's review of the **conformation**, or structure, of your dog's body. Conformation includes the shape and angle of your dog's bones and joints, as well as your dog's overall body condition. (Abnormal **angulation** of bones or joints greatly increases a dog's risk of osteoarthritis.) Next, your veterinarian will carefully observe your dog as he rises, sits, and walks. Your veterinarian should also perform **palpation** (examination with the hands) of your dog's body for muscle **atrophy** or weakness and joint **effusion** (swelling with fluid). Finally, your veterinarian will palpate all bones and move the joints to determine your dog's range of motion and to detect any pain and **crepitus** (a subtle grinding found with the bony changes of osteoarthritis).

Examination of the arthritic dog may show these problems:

- **Muscle atrophy (deterioration)**
- **Joint swelling or fibrosis (excessive formation of scar-type tissue)**
- **Decreased range of motion of a joint**
- **Pain and crepitus when a joint is moved and manipulated**

# Radiography

Often the next step in the diagnosis of osteoarthritis is **radiography**, or x-ray examination. Your dog may be sedated for x-ray studies, partly because the quality of the radiographs is better when your dog lies still and partly because sedation will lessen any stress and pain that your dog might experience during the procedure. Sedation also allows the veterinarian to palpate your dog more thoroughly and to determine exactly where pain is occurring. There is very little risk associated with sedation of your dog.

Osteoarthritis is often accompanied by an increase in **joint fluid** and thickening of the soft tissue of the joint capsule. Joint fluid and soft tissue, which both appear dark on x-rays, may be seen in larger amounts on these images.

In osteoarthritis, the cartilage of the joint is the part that is affected the most. As osteoarthritis gets worse and the cartilage becomes thinner, the bone underlying the diseased cartilage reacts to this loss of cushioning by becoming harder, or **sclerotic**. On x-rays, the areas of **sclerosis** usually appear as increased whiteness of the bone next to the joint.

One of the most common signs of osteoarthritis seen on an x-ray is **osteophytosis**. As osteoarthritis gets worse, the dog's body creates nodules of bone at the edges of the joint. These nodules or bumps, called **osteo-**

**phytes**, show up on the x-ray as new, irregularly shaped bone. Although they almost never affect the dog's joint function or **range of motion,** they do indicate that the disease is chronic and severe.

Radiography is the most commonly used and easily available test for the diagnosis of osteoarthritis, but vet-

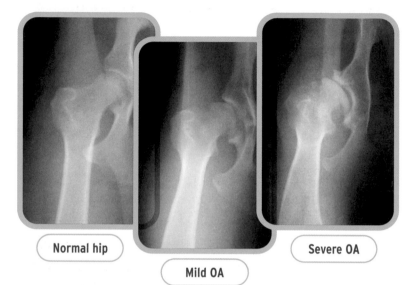

Normal hip

Mild OA

Severe OA

erinarians and dog owners must keep in mind that x-rays have their limitations. Cartilage cannot be seen on radiographs, so it is impossible to learn from an x-ray whether cartilage is damaged and, if it is, how much so. With the ever-increasing development of canine arthroscopy (discussed later in this chapter), the limitations of radiography to diagnose osteoarthritis have become clearer. Recent studies have shown that radiographs do not do a good job of showing the condition of cartilage. In fact, dogs with very few signs of osteoarthritis on x-rays were often found to have a lot of damage to the cartilage of the elbow or hip when the veterinarian performed arthroscopy later.

To get an accurate radiographic diagnosis of osteoarthritis, your veterinarian (or a specialist in veterinary radiography) must use high-quality x-rays and must either be experienced at reading and evaluating radiographs or send them to someone who is. Even under these conditions, problems with the cartilage in a joint may not be easy to detect on a radiograph. Ultimately the only way your veterinarian can determine the condition of the cartilage is to look at it directly through the use of **arthrotomy** (open-joint surgery) or **arthroscopy** (in which a small illuminated imaging tool known as an **endoscope** is inserted through a small cut in the joint).

# Joint Fluid Analysis

Your veterinarian may analyze the fluid in a joint to diagnose osteoarthritis and other joint diseases. A needle is inserted into the joint to obtain the fluid, in a procedure called **arthrocentesis**. Usually the dog is sedated; then the fur around the joint is clipped and the skin is scrubbed to lower the risk of infection. It's not always easy to obtain joint fluid because a joint may contain only a small amount of it. (A small volume of fluid can be a good sign because it shows that more serious problems, such as infection or immune joint disease, are less likely.) Your veterinarian usually cannot tell by analyzing the joint fluid what is causing the osteoarthritis, but analysis is a valuable tool when there is a question about the diagnosis.

# Arthroscopy

Arthroscopy—inserting an endoscope into a small cut to help see and treat a joint—does require general anesthesia, but it is much less invasive than arthrotomy (surgically opening the joint). The technique is less stressful for your dog, so your veterinarian may perform arthroscopy of several joints in one procedure. In most cases arthroscopy shows the inside of a joint much better than arthrotomy does.

Veterinarians also use arthroscopy to treat joints. As these techniques become more advanced and as more surgeons learn to use them, arthroscopy is becoming the standard treatment for many joint diseases in dogs.

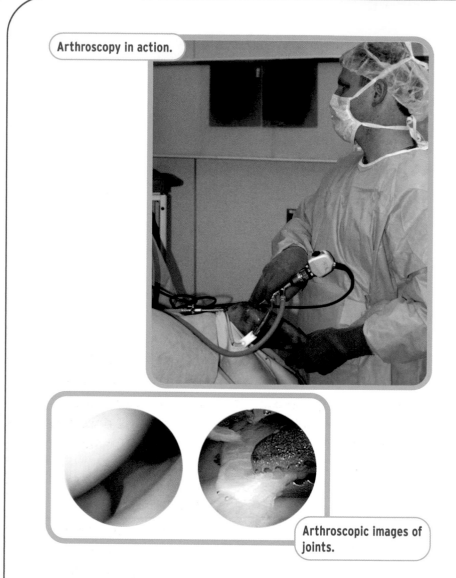

Arthroscopy in action.

Arthroscopic images of joints.

# Other Tools

## Magnetic Resonance Imaging (MRI)

**Magnetic resonance imaging**, or MRI, has been used in veterinary surgery for many years now, mostly to help veterinarians see soft tissue diseases. Although MRI has been used for years to diagnose human joint diseases, it has not been as useful in dogs, mainly because of the size of the patient and the thickness of the cartilage. Canine

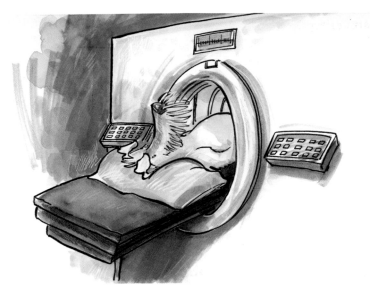

cartilage is much thinner than human cartilage, so MRI for dogs requires powerful machines and long exposure times, plus general anesthesia. MRI may become more valuable in the imaging of cartilage in dogs, but right now it's used mostly to see the ligaments and tendons surrounding joints.

## Computed Tomography (CT)

**Computed tomography**, or CT, is valuable to veterinarians because it helps them see the bone around a joint. It's also been used to examine fractures and the developmental diseases of the joints that occur when a dog has poor conformation. Because cartilage doesn't show up on CT scans, CT really can't be used to look at cartilage damage caused by osteoarthritis. As with MRI, a dog that undergoes CT must have general anesthesia.

## Ultrasound Examination

Veterinarians sometimes use **ultrasonography**, or **ultrasound examination**, to evaluate joints. Ultrasonography *is* useful in helping the veterinarian evaluate the soft tis-

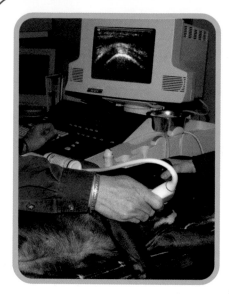

sues surrounding a dog's joints, especially the shoulder, where ligament or tendon injury may cause osteoarthritis. Usually during an ultrasound examination the dog is awake or lightly sedated.

## Bone Scanning

In a **bone scan**, low-level radioactivity is used to show parts of the skeleton with increased blood supply and bone **turnover** (the body's way of maintaining bone strength), which are signs of diseases such as osteoarthritis.

Before the scan, a radioactive agent that accumulates quickly in bone is injected into the dog's vein. The skeleton is photographed with a special camera that "sees" the radiation. Increased radioactivity in a particular area may indicate osteoarthritis. The bone scan is safe for your dog (and you), but the dog usually has to stay in the hospital for a day or two.

Your veterinarian will not be able to diagnose osteoarthritis just by looking at a bone scan, but the scan may show the location of disease. Bone scans are most useful when the veterinarian is having trouble finding the source of pain or lameness. Most of the time, bone scanning is performed while the dog is awake or perhaps under light sedation.

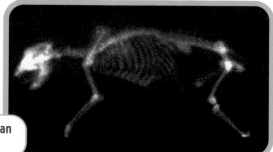

Whole body bone scan of dog.

Now let's review the information in this chapter:

■ A proper evaluation for osteoarthritis includes the dog's history (the signs and problems you have noticed), a general physical examination, and an orthopedic examination.

■ Palpating (using the hands to examine) your dog's limbs is the single most important method used by the veterinarian to look for osteoarthritis and other joint diseases.

■ During the orthopedic examination of a dog with osteoarthritis, the veterinarian may find muscle atrophy (degeneration), joint swelling, less range of motion, and pain when the arthritic joint is moved.

■ Radiographs (x-rays) of a dog with osteoarthritis may show increased joint fluid, bone hardening (sclerosis), and new bone formation (osteophytosis).

■ Your veterinarian may also use joint-fluid analysis, arthroscopy, MRI (magnetic-resonance imaging), CT (computed tomography), ultrasound, or nuclear bone scanning to diagnose osteoarthritis in your dog.

# PART TWO

# Treatment of Osteoarthritis

Osteoarthritis treatment is usually divided into surgical and medical categories, although your veterinarian may combine the two approaches for the best possible treatment. Medical management is also referred to as "conservative" or "nonsurgical" treatment. The terminology can be confusing, especially because "medical" management is much more than just the use of medications. In fact, sometimes prescription drugs are not used at all.

The medical management of osteoarthritis is based on five principles: weight management, use of nutritional supplements, exercise, physical rehabilitation, and anti-inflammatory therapy. These topics are covered in Chapters 5 through 9. Most of these principles are interrelated: Exercise and nutrition are important parts of weight management, and exercise is a major component of physical rehabilitation. Still, not all of these therapies are used in every case of canine osteoarthritis.

In addition to medical management, your veterinarian may use surgery to treat osteoarthritis. Surgery of the joints and bones is part of the specialty called **orthopedic surgery**. Your veterinarian can choose from many procedures to restore function to your dog's joints. Osteoarthritis surgery is the topic of Chapter 10.

Alternative therapies such as acupuncture are also available for dogs with osteoarthritis. Such therapies for osteoarthritis are covered in Chapter 11.

## The Five Principles of the Medical Management of Osteoarthritis

★ PRINCIPLE **1**  Weight management
★ PRINCIPLE **2**  Use of nutritional supplements
★ PRINCIPLE **3**  Appropriate exercise
★ PRINCIPLE **4**  Physical rehabilitation
★ PRINCIPLE **5**  Medications

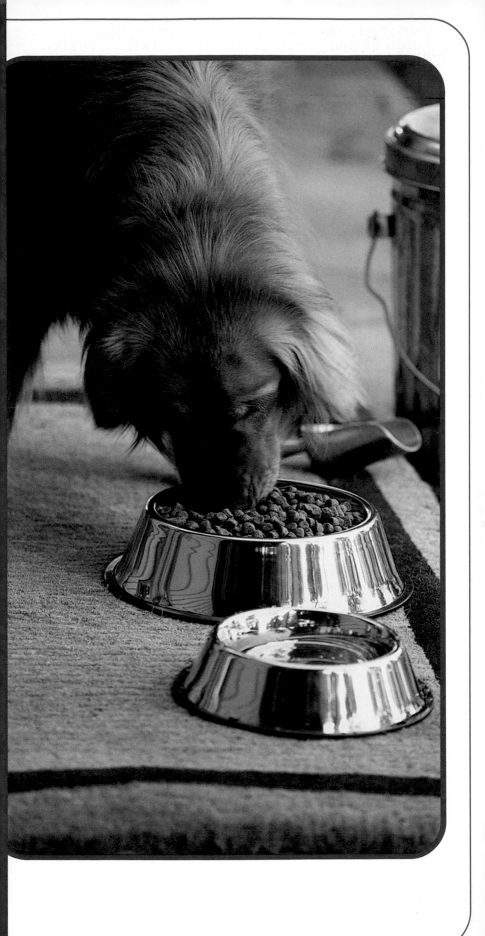

# Body Weight Management

**PRINCIPLE 1**

Being overweight is the main factor that makes the signs of osteoarthritis worse and causes arthritis to get worse faster. You may be able to reduce or even get rid of the need for costly and risky medications and surgeries by helping your dog lose excess weight and maintain a healthy weight. A thin dog with osteoarthritis will feel better and will be more active than an overweight one, and the thinner dog is also likely to live longer. This chapter shows you how to find out whether your dog is overweight and how to work with your veterinarian to come up with a diet that will give your dog the best possible quality of life.

# Benefits of Healthy Weight

Keeping your dog at a healthy weight has several important benefits:

- You may be able to delay or even prevent the need for expensive surgery.
- Your dog may no longer need pain medications or may need less of these drugs.
- Your dog's quality of life will be improved.
- Your dog may live longer.

## Where We Stand

Getting your dog down to the proper weight is the single most important thing *you* can do to prevent or treat your dog's osteoarthritis.

# Body Weight and Osteoarthritis

The load on joints during everyday activity changes with your dog's weight. As your dog's weight increases, so do the forces exerted on cartilage, bone, and soft tissues. As weight decreases, the forces decrease. This is especially important in joints with osteoarthritis. By decreasing the amount of force on a joint, we can slow down the degeneration and ease the day-to-day pain of osteoarthritis.

In dogs with osteoarthritis of the hip joints (which is usually caused by hip dysplasia), it has been shown that weight loss brings real relief of **lameness** and pain. In many cases the effect of weight loss is so dramatic that surgery is no longer needed and the pain medications are

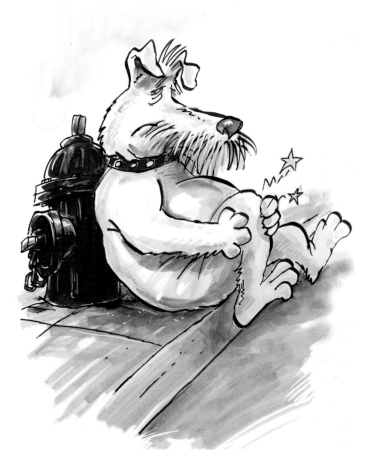

cut back or even stopped. Food restriction, weight loss, and good body condition will make your dog more comfortable and more willing to exercise and will decrease the need for medication if your dog has osteoarthritis. This information should be a strong incentive for the owner of a dog with osteoarthritis to adopt a weight-loss program that will help the dog achieve a healthy weight.

# Role of Nutrition

Health and nutrition are directly related. People who eat poorly are often obese and are more likely to have heart disease or **diabetes.** A dog fed a poor diet may have similar diseases, but it's interesting to note that dogs are actually fed better, more balanced diets than many people eat. Dogs in our society are fortunate because many improvements in canine nutrition have been made over the past 50 years. The importance of dogs in many roles—family members, companions, athletes, workers—has stimulated research into dogs' nutritional needs. Your dog's diet is important in preventing illness *and* in treating many diseases. The combinations of ingredients in high-quality dog foods are based on years of scientific research involving veterinarians and dog owners. Feeding your dog the proper food in the proper amount has tremendous health benefits.

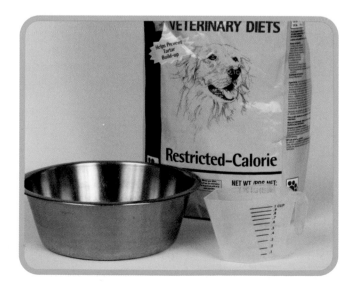

Despite all this progress, dog owners still find that their pets experience dietary problems, especially being overweight. These problems have several causes:

- **A diet too high in calories**
- **Too much dog food**
- **Too much human food**
- **Too many high-calorie treats**

# Body Weight and Body Condition Scoring

So how do we decide if a dog is overweight and by how much? Veterinarians do this by determining a dog's **body**

## Nestlé PURINA
## BODY CONDITION SYSTEM

**TOO THIN**

**1**   Ribs, lumbar vertebrae, pelvic bones and all bony prominences evident from a distance. No discernible body fat. Obvious loss of muscle mass.

**2**   Ribs, lumbar vertebrae and pelvic bones easily visible. No palpable fat. Some evidence of other bony prominence. Minimal loss of muscle mass.

**3**   Ribs easily palpated and may be visible with no palpable fat. Tops of lumbar vertebrae visible. Pelvic bones becoming prominent. Obvious waist and abdominal tuck.

**IDEAL**

**4**   Ribs easily palpable, with minimal fat covering. Waist easily noted, viewed from above. Abdominal tuck evident.

**5**   Ribs palpable without excess fat covering. Waist observed behind ribs when viewed from above. Abdomen tucked up when viewed from side.

**TOO HEAVY**

**6**   Ribs palpable with slight excess fat covering. Waist is discernible viewed from above but is not prominent. Abdominal tuck apparent.

**7**   Ribs palpable with difficulty; heavy fat cover. Noticeable fat deposits over lumbar area and base of tail. Waist absent or barely visible. Abdominal tuck may be present.

**8**   Ribs not palpable under very heavy fat cover, or palpable only with significant pressure. Heavy fat deposits over lumbar area and base of tail. Waist absent. No abdominal tuck. Obvious abdominal distention may be present.

**9**   Massive fat deposits over thorax, spine and base of tail. Waist and abdominal tuck absent. Fat deposits on neck and limbs. Obvious abdominal distention.

The **BODY CONDITION SYSTEM** was developed at the Nestlé Purina Pet Care Center and has been validated as documented in the following publications:

Mawby D, Bartges JW, Moyers T, et. al. *Comparison of body fat estimates by dual-energy x-ray absorptiometry and deuterium oxide dilution in client owned dogs.* Compendium 2001; 23 (9A): 70

LaFlamme DP. *Development and Validation of a Body Condition Score System for Dogs.* Canine Practice July/August 1997; 22:10-15

Kealy, et. al. *Effects of Diet Restriction on Life Span and Age-Related Changes in Dogs.* JAVMA 2002; 220:1315-1320

**Call 1-800-222-VETS (8387), weekdays, 8:00 a.m. to 4:30 p.m. CT**

## Nestlé PURINA

75

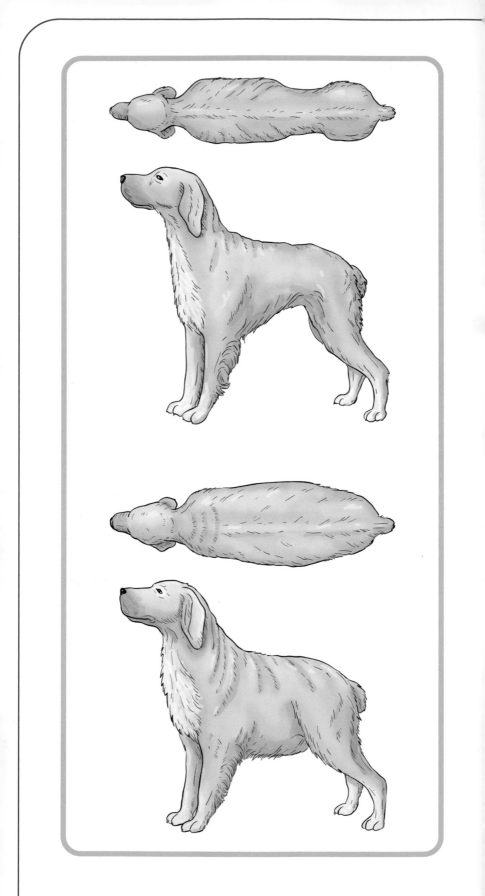

**condition score**, or BCS. The BCS is a scale of 1 to 9 (some veterinarians use a 1 to 5 scale) that's used to judge the dog's appearance and the amount of fat on its body (see Appendix A). A BCS of 4 or 5 is considered normal and healthy, a BCS of 1 shows that a dog is severely underweight, and a dog with a BCS of 9 is obese. You can also get a rough estimate of appropriate weight by considering the dog's breed, but the BCS system is a much better way to judge a dog's weight. (A table of appropriate body weights for different breeds of dogs is provided in Appendix B.)

# Starting a Weight-Loss Program

Just as in people, the first step in a weight-loss program for your dog is an honest, accurate assessment of body condition. Getting your veterinarian involved at this point is important. The veterinarian will perform a complete physical examination and may recommend blood work to find out if your dog has other medical diseases or conditions that make losing weight difficult. A low-calorie diet is not recommended in dogs with certain medical diseases and could endanger your pet's overall health. Also, **hypothyroidism** (too-low levels of thyroid hormones) makes weight loss difficult. Fortunately, your veterinarian can treat this disease using supplementary thyroid hormones.

The following information is required to start a weight-loss program for your dog:

- **Initial body weight**
- **Starting BCS (Body Condition Score)**
- **Target body weight**
- **Target BCS**
- **Daily calorie allowance**

You should get help from your veterinarian to accurately weigh your pet, determine the starting BCS, and find a target weight and BCS.

As the most qualified person to guide you, your veterinarian will help obtain the information needed to begin the program and assess your dog throughout the program until the target weight is reached. You should consider monthly trips to your veterinary clinic for reweighing, reassessment of your pet's BCS, and fine-tuning of the calories your pet eats each day. University studies have shown that the most important factor in the success of a weight loss program is *regular follow-up* to weigh the dog and evaluate progress. You and your veterinarian should aim to get your dog to his target weight within 12 to 20 weeks. The more weight your dog needs to lose, the longer it will take to get to the target weight. Helping your dog lose weight is challenging, but with your veterinarian's advice and encouragement, your pet's goal weight can be reached.

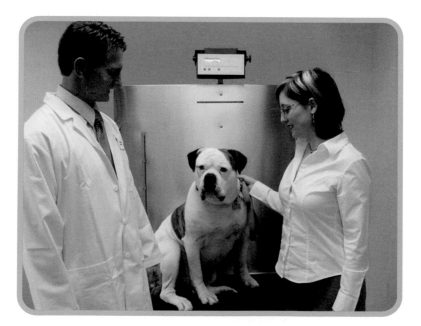

# Nestlé Purina Labrador Retriever Lifetime Study

Recently the Pet Nutrition Department of the Nestlé Purina Co. completed a 15-year study of a group of 48 Labrador retrievers. The study was designed to determine the effect of diet on the lifespan of dogs and the severity of osteoarthritis. Half of the dogs were allowed to eat as much food as they liked. The other 24 dogs were allowed to eat just 75% of what the first group ate. The results of this study were dramatic, and they greatly increased the understanding of the effect of diet on lifespan and osteoarthritis in dogs.

## Weight and Life Expectancy

The dogs that were fed a low-calorie diet lived, on average, 22 months longer than the dogs in the study that got 25% more food each day. The dogs given less food also had a lower incidence and later onset of chronic disease. From these findings it is clear that maintaining a healthy body condition can lengthen your dog's lifespan.

## Weight and Osteoarthritis

In the Nestlé Purina Labrador Retriever Lifetime Study, the mean weight of the dogs in the group fed a low-calorie diet was 25% less than that of the overfed dogs. This difference translates to a much lighter load on the joints over a dog's lifespan. Osteoarthritis was more likely in the dogs given more food; it developed earlier in these dogs' lives and was more severe as well. These dogs required more medication to control the pain of osteoarthritis and were less able to get around than the dogs fed fewer calories. In the dogs maintained at a mean weight 25% less than that of their overweight counterparts, the risk of osteoarthritis was lower and the disease was less severe when it did occur. Again, this study shows that maintaining your dog at its proper weight can have tremendous effects on its quality of life by reducing the severity and pain of osteoarthritis.

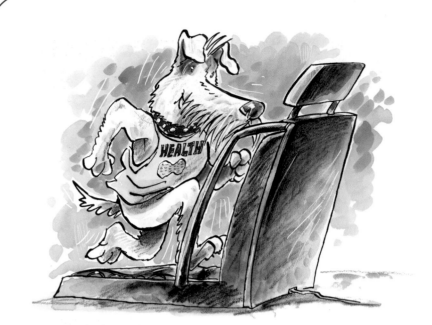

## Choosing an Ideal Weight

Figuring out your dog's ideal weight is not easy. It requires the help of someone with experience, especially because the ideal may need to be adjusted as your dog loses weight. A BCS of 4 or 5 (on that scale of 1 to 9) is the goal. Each point your dog is above the ideal BCS means your dog is overweight by an additional 10%. So a dog with a BCS of 8 is 30% overweight if we use 5 as a goal and 40% overweight if we use 4 as a goal ($8 - 4 = 4 \rightarrow 4 \times 10 = 40\%$).

The goal of a weight-loss plan is to achieve the target weight within 12 to 20 weeks, or to lose 1% to 2% of the dog's weight each week.

## Calculating Ideal Body Weight from BCS Score

You can estimate the percentage of body weight that your dog should lose by subtracting the goal BCS from the current BCS. Every 1-point difference between the present and target BCS (on the 1 to 9 scale) indicates that your dog needs to lose about 10% of its total weight.

For example, Fido weighs 88 lb and has a BCS of 8. His target BCS is 4, which represents his best body condition. Fido needs to lose 4 BCS points. If each BCS point represents 10% of total body weight, Fido should lose about 40% of his total body weight, or 35 lb. You and your veterinarian would then set Fido's goal weight at 53 lb.

## Figuring Daily Calorie Requirements

The number of calories your dog can eat each day and still reach the target weight and BCS is based on a dietary value called the **resting energy requirement**, or RER. The RER is simply the number of calories a dog at a specific weight requires each day. (A table of RER data is provided in Appendix C.) **Remember, you base the number of calories your dog needs on the ideal weight, not on the dog's current weight!** In some cases the number of calo-

## How Calorie Needs Are Calculated

Every dog has a resting energy requirement, or RER. This calculation is based on the energy requirements of a dog with a low activity level, and this is the reason for the "resting" in the name. Although you may consider your dog active or you may be increasing the dog's activity to help her lose weight, don't use this as an excuse to feed her more than the RER. Feeding the RER for the desired weight is almost always more than enough to help an overweight dog lose weight. You may feel as if you're starving your dog on this diet, but you're actually providing plenty of calories. Besides, your dog has all that extra fat to burn off!

The RER information in Appendix C was calculated using this formula:

Calories = $70 \times$ (kilograms of body weight)$^{0.75}$

This formula is accepted by dietary scientists and veterinarians as the best way to determine a dog's caloric needs.

ries may be more or less than the RER, but almost always you can help your dog lose enough weight in a reasonable amount of time by feeding the RER of the desired weight.

Once the ideal or target weight and BCS are reached, you can feed your pet at the RER of that weight and maintain his ideal weight and condition.

The idea of appropriate daily calorie intake is not hard to understand, but mistakes in these calculations will make it harder for your dog to lose weight and may even lead to harm. Have your veterinarian perform these calculations to make sure that the daily calorie recommendation is accurate.

As we mentioned earlier, the RER is the *resting* energy requirement—the energy required for a less active dog at a certain body weight or an overweight dog trying to reach that body weight. Sometimes the RER is used only as a starting point. For instance:

- Your veterinarian may recommend feeding just 80% of the RER in an overweight dog that isn't losing enough weight.
- Your veterinarian may tell you to feed more than the RER if your dog weighs what it should and is an active athlete or a working dog.
- If you are using the RER system to feed your dog, check with your veterinarian before making any long-term changes.

## Food Types and Caloric Densities

Every dog food, dry or canned, has a specific caloric density—the number of calories present in a certain weight or volume of the food. Reputable dog food manufacturers make this information freely available to the pet owner. Dog foods for weight loss are available at grocery stores, pet supply stores, and your veterinary clinic. Sometimes the ingredients of diets from your veterinarian are similar to those sold in stores, but often the "veterinary" diet is more specialized. Some important information on the contents of many of the "veterinary" diets is shown in Appendix D.

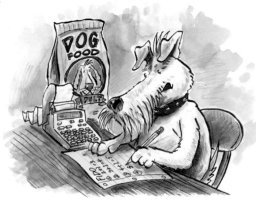

## Fido's Diet

Let's say that Fido, our cartoon dog, weighs 80 lb, but we have decided with the help of our veterinarian that he should weigh 65 lb. Looking at the RER chart in Appendix C, we see that a dog weighing 65 lb should normally consume about 900 calories a day (887, to be exact). This daily calorie intake includes *everything*, including any treats or human food that Fido might get. (By the way, we don't really encourage the feeding of people food or table scraps to your dog. People food tends to be high in calories, and owners often don't account for it in the daily calorie intake.)

This may not look like a lot of food, but Fido's not starving—he just thinks he is. There are many tricks you can use to keep Fido (and you, his owner) happy, eliminate Fido's constant feeling of hunger, and ease your feelings of guilt while keeping Fido's weight loss on track.

Every few weeks or so, Fido visits the veterinary clinic, where he can be weighed on the same scale every time and the vet can assess progress. The goal here is to lose 1% to 2% of body weight per week—in Fido's case, 1 to 1.5 lb. If Fido isn't making progress, his owner and the veterinarian should determine whether the diet is being followed. If weight loss is too slow, Fido's veterinarian may recommend feeding only 80% of Fido's RER. If weight loss is too rapid—this is rare—the veterinarian may recommend giving Fido a little more food.

Regular follow-up with the veterinarian and sticking strictly to the diet will help Fido reach his target weight in just a few short months.

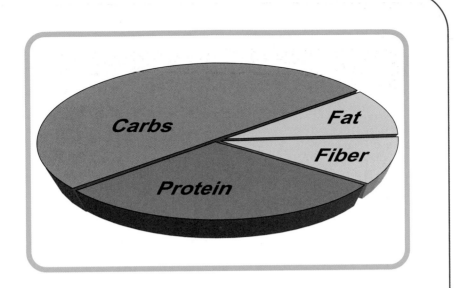

Commercial dog foods, which are made from many plant and animal sources, contain certain percentages of **carbohydrate,** protein, fat, fiber, moisture, vitamins, and minerals. Reputable companies have veterinary nutritionists create balanced foods with appropriate levels of protein, carbohydrate, fat, and nutrients.

Low-calorie dog foods for weight loss or weight control often contain 200 to 300 calories per cup. Once you have chosen a food and identified its caloric density, you can easily figure out how much food to feed each day: Just divide your dog's daily caloric need by the caloric density of the food.

# Tips and Strategies for Weight Loss

You can give your dog the total daily ration of dog food in the morning or serve several smaller meals during the day. The most important thing to remember: Do NOT exceed the total daily food allowance.

At night your dog can have a small bowl of plain steamed or microwaved vegetables. This will give your dog extra fiber without a lot of extra calories. Try serving spinach, green beans, peas, carrots, broccoli, or cauliflower. Never feed your dog starchy carbohydrates such as potatoes, rice, bread, or other baked goods; they're high in calories. If your dog is used to getting treats, try baby carrots or cut-up apples. Never give your dog calorie-rich treats, chews, or marrow bones if you are trying to help your dog lose weight.

## A Note about Treats

Treats can be a major obstacle to dieting for your dog. Often they're high in calories, and many dog owners don't even count them in the daily calorie intake. But dogs love treats, and owners (and children) love to give them to their pets, so here are some tips to help your dog stay on its diet and still get special treats now and then:

1. Limit the number of treats you give your dog each day, and be sure that everyone in the family agrees on this limit.
2. Look for low-calorie dog treats.
3. Try using rice cakes as treats.
4. Dogs love carrots, which are very low in calories.

Keeping your dog out of the kitchen and dining area while you and your family prepare and eat meals may be helpful. Dogs have a keen sense of smell, and the aromas of cooking will stimulate your pet's appetite. If you can manage it, choose one person in the family to be in charge of your dog's feeding and diet to make sure that your pet is getting the right foods in the right amounts,

You should also start your dog on a program of mild to moderate exercise. Incorporating these diet and exercise recommendations into your dog's lifestyle will help your pet maintain an ideal weight and overall health.

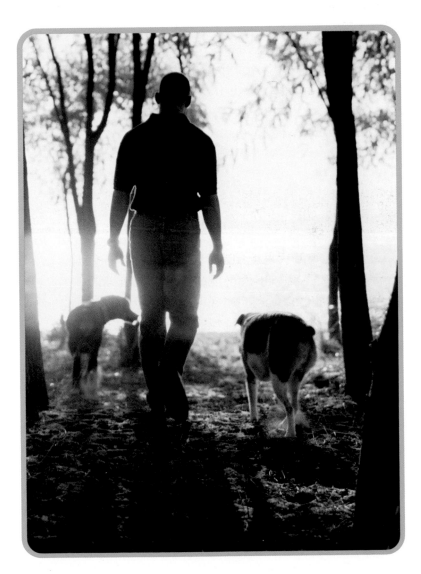

## The Seven Steps of a Weight-Loss Program

1. Work with your veterinarian to determine your dog's BCS.
2. Figure out your dog's ideal weight.
3. Calculate the daily calories (RER) to achieve the desired BCS and weight.
4. Find out the caloric density of your dog food.
5. Figure out how much to feed your dog each day. Don't forget to include treats in total calories.
6. Remember, exercise is important.
7. Have your dog weighed at least once every 4 weeks, and regulate the amount of food you give your dog to be sure that it loses 1% or 2% of its weight each week.

Developing a successful weight-loss program and sticking to a feeding plan will be challenging for you *and* your dog. To guarantee the success of your program, you need to accurately assess your dog's current weight and BCS, review your feeding practices, and adopt a healthy, realistic feeding plan that you will adhere to for the long term. Adhering to a weight-loss program will reduce the pain of osteoarthritis and give your dog a dramatically improved quality of life.

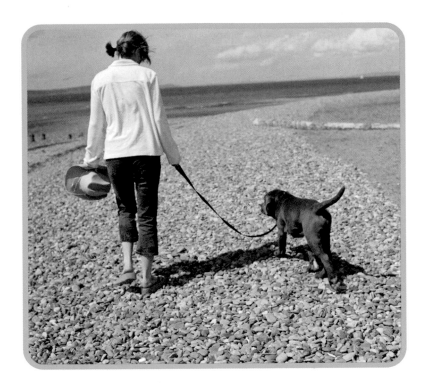

Now let's review the information in this chapter:

- **Controlling your dog's weight is the single most effective way you can improve your dog's quality of life.**
- **Many dogs in the United States are overweight.**
- **Weight loss is usually simple and inexpensive; only the willpower of the owner is required.**
- **The Body Condition Score system is used to judge a dog's body weight.**
- **In the most common weight-loss diet for dogs, the overweight dog is fed 80% to 100% of the calorie requirements of the ideal body weight (RER).**
- **Regular follow-up with your veterinarian is the most important way to guarantee the success of a weight-loss program for your dog.**

# CHAPTER 6

**PRINCIPLE 2**

# Nutritional Supplements

In this chapter we look at the main nutritional supplements for dogs, how they work, and how to find a reputable source. There are hundreds of nutritional supplements on the market for the treatment of osteoarthritis. Unfortunately, most of them have never really been tested to show whether they actually help dogs with osteoarthritis. Some of these products may be dangerous, and many are expensive. Research is beginning to show which supplements are effective and which are not. You, as the consumer, need a source of information to help decide which products are worth purchasing and which manufacturers can be trusted.

# Development of Nutritional Supplements

The use of nutritional supplements for the treatment of osteoarthritis in dogs has become extremely popular. Unfortunately, the science of this field is still young, and there is a lot of misinformation about it. There are major problems with the quality and reliability of these products, and that means that the buyer must beware. In spite of these problems, the potential benefits and the general low risk of side effects of good-quality ingredients suggest that some of these products may be helpful to dogs with osteoarthritis. Supplements are available in specially made dog foods (called "therapeutic diets") designed for dogs with osteoarthritis, or they can be found as separate

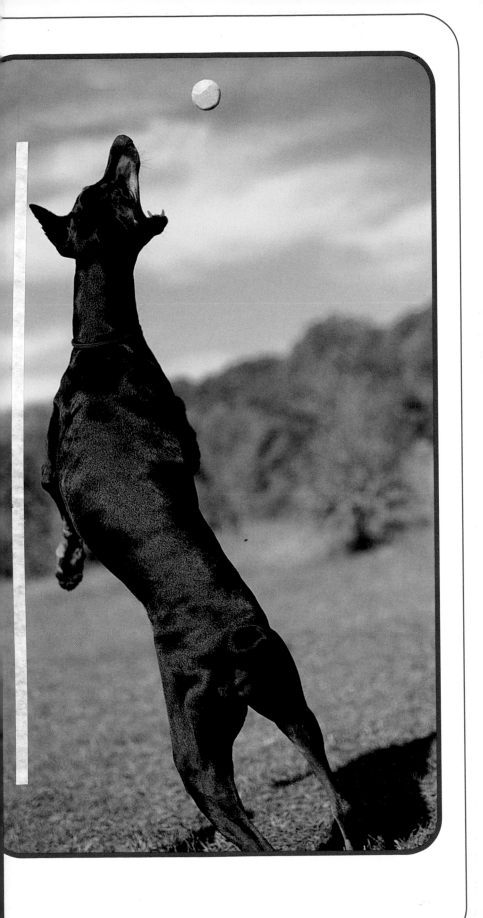

products that you can give your dog. Some supplements, such as **omega-3 fatty acids,** are found naturally in a dog's diet, but the amount or specific type of supplement may be changed when your dog is being treated for osteoarthritis. Other products, such as **glucosamine** and chondroitin, are found only in small amounts in a dog's diet. These fall into the category known as nutraceuticals.

# What Are Nutraceuticals?

"Nutraceutical" is a term taken from the words "nutrition" and "pharmaceutical." The term **nutraceutical** is technically defined by the North American Veterinary Nutraceutical Council as "a nondrug substance that is produced in a purified or extracted form and administered orally to provide agents required for normal body structure and function with the intent of improving the health and well-being of animals." What this means is that they are naturally occurring products that are eaten to improve health. Not all nutraceuticals are used to treat osteoarthritis. It's been suggested that nutraceuticals can be used to treat liver and heart disease and to benefit the skin and coat of dogs as well.

# What Supplements Are Used to Treat Osteoarthritis?

The list of supplements that manufacturers have claimed are useful in the treatment of osteoarthritis is long. The most common ones are:

- **Omega-3 fatty acids**
- **Glucosamine**
- **Chondroitin sulfate**
- **Vitamin C**
- **Methylsulfonylmethane (MSM)**

- *Perna canaliculus* (green-lipped) mussel
- Other antioxidants

These compounds generally fall into one or both of the following categories:

1. Those that may positively affect cartilage metabolism
2. Those that may have "natural" anti-inflammatory properties

As we've discussed before, the actual science of nutritional supplements for osteoarthritis lags far behind the advertising and marketing of these supplements. In this chapter we'll discuss only the supplements about which there is reliable information. We recommend that you use only supplements that contain products we believe will benefit your dog in the treatment of osteoarthritis.

# Does My Dog Need Supplements?

In our veterinary practices, we recommend nutritional supplements for many of our patients with osteoarthritis.

Why? The right supplements may help ease the pain of osteoarthritis. Although nutritional supplements can't cure **arthritis** and may not be helpful in all cases, most of them are safe. Also, evidence suggests that when people use nutritional supplements, it can lessen the need for anti-inflammatory drugs. Consult with your regular veterinarian or veterinary surgeon about the use of these supplements. Your veterinarian can help you balance the use of these products with the other four principles in the medical management of osteoarthritis (listed in Chapter 5). We recognize the high cost and the potential problems with product quality, so we do not recommend supplements arbitrarily.

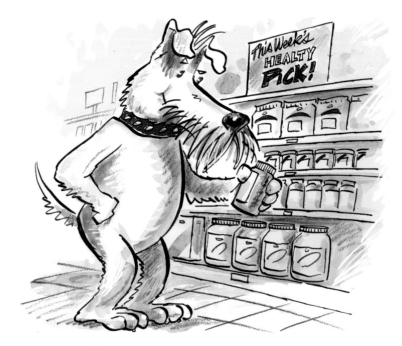

# How Do Supplements Work?

Some supplements used experimentally under laboratory conditions do help form new cartilage, and this same effect may also happen in dogs. However, it's more likely

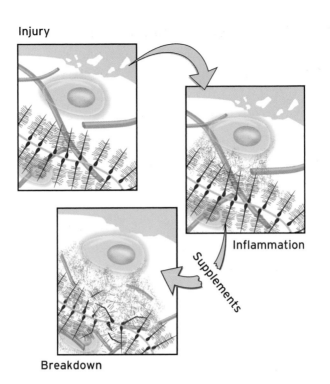

Injury

Inflammation

Supplements

Breakdown

that nutritional supplements work primarily to help decrease the inflammation in the joints that makes cartilage damage worse and increases the pain of osteoarthritis. Various supplements have other effects, which are described later on.

True cartilage healing most often happens when the cartilage has been damaged but the underlying conformation or structure of the joint is normal—for instance, in the case of a fracture involving the joint, or a torn **ligament.** When the joint can be restored to normal, the cartilage is likely to heal to its near-normal condition, and nutritional supplements may aid in this type of healing.

Unfortunately, most osteoarthritis in dogs is associated with underlying abnormalities of the joint, such as **dysplasia** or chronically weak ligaments. In these cases the cartilage is not likely to heal because the mechanical forces—the abnormalities—working to destroy the cartilage are much greater than the biological forces that are working to heal it. Nutritional supplements may help quite

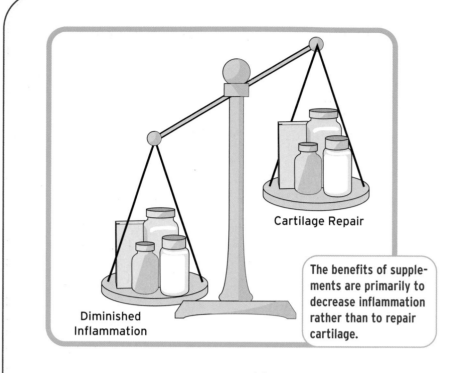

Cartilage Repair

The benefits of supplements are primarily to decrease inflammation rather than to repair cartilage.

Diminished Inflammation

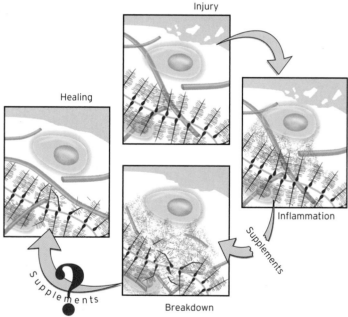

Injury

Healing

Inflammation

Supplements

Breakdown

Supplements

a bit in these cases anyway, though, because their anti-inflammatory properties may help ease the pain.

## What Are Omega-3 Fatty Acids?

No doubt you have seen many different and confusing names for these supplements. Some of these names are:

- **Long-chain omega-3 polyunsaturated fatty acids**
- **Omega-3 fatty acids**
- **Eicosapentaenoic acid, or EPA**
- **Docosahexaenoic acid, or DHA**
- **Dietary *n*-3 fatty acids**
- **Fish oil supplements**

Omega-3 fatty acids have many health benefits. Apparently, if they are given in the correct dosages, they act as an anti-inflammatory. Omega-3 fatty acids work by replacing an element in the cell walls—**arachidonic acid, or AA**—with a different element—eicosapentaenoic acid, or EPA. When a joint is injured, AA breaks down into chemicals that increase pain and inflammation. On the other hand, when EPA breaks down after an injury it produces chemicals that are less inflammatory and even potentially anti-inflammatory. Replacing AA with EPA decreases the pain and inflammation associated with joint injury or os-

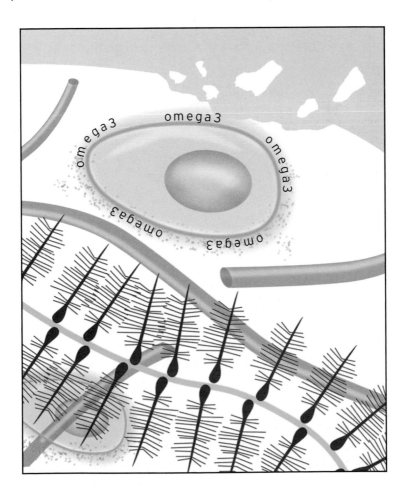

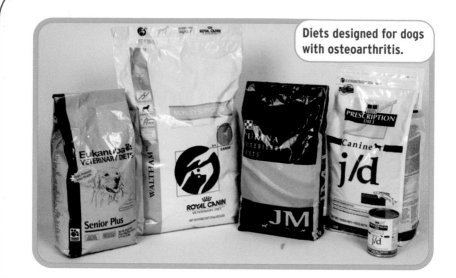

Diets designed for dogs with osteoarthritis.

teoarthritis. Omega-3 fatty acids may also help ease inflammation by blocking some of the genes that cause inflammation in osteoarthritis.

### How Are Omega-3 Fatty Acids Administered?

Omega-3 fatty acids may be administered either in a commercial dog food made especially for dogs with osteoarthritis or as individual supplements, such as fish oil capsules. Several major dog food companies make diets for dogs with osteoarthritis. These diets usually include omega-3 fatty acids and may also include glucosamine and chondroitin. Some of these diets are low-calorie to help dogs lose weight (see Appendix E).

## Where We Stand

Current evidence on the use of omega-3 fatty acids in the management of osteoarthritis in dogs is promising. We recommend the use of a specially formulated "osteoarthritis diet" or proper dietary supplementation with omega-3 fatty acids for most of our patients with osteoarthritis.

### Are Omega-3 Fatty Acids Effective?

Studies in dogs have suggested that omega-3 fatty acids can ease the pain of osteoarthritis. In one study, about 80% of the dogs studied showed improved function when they were fed diets that included omega-3 fatty acids. These findings are based on what the owners observed, what the veterinarians observed, and a computer analysis of the dogs' leg function. It's also been shown in both humans and dogs that including omega-3 fatty acids in the diet can decrease the need for **NSAIDs (non-steroidal anti-inflammatory drugs),** such as aspirin and

## Should I Use a Therapeutic Food or Individual Supplements to Provide My Dog with Omega-3 Fatty Acids?

Fatty acids may be provided either in a dog food with omega-3 fatty acids specifically included or in supplements that provide only fatty acids. Either method is acceptable. A therapeutic dog food is usually more convenient, but if you cannot or do not want to switch dog foods, consider supplementation. The relative cost depends on the dog food or supplement you select, but some estimates are provided below. Adding these also adds fat and therefore calories.

| Feature | Arthritis Diet (4 cups) | Omega-3 Supplement | | |
| --- | --- | --- | --- | --- |
| | | 1 | 2 | 3 |
| Omega-3 content | 1600 mg/ meal | 180 mg/ capsule | 250 mg/ capsule | 100 mg/ pump |
| Equivalent amounts | 4 cups | 9 capsules | 6 capsules | 13 pumps |
| Cost per day | 1.45 | 0.75 plus regular dog food | 1.00 plus regular dog food | 1.57 plus regular dog food |

Rimadyl. The scientific evidence supporting the use of omega-3 fatty acids is strong and growing. More studies need to be done, but because this supplement is generally safe and useful, it can be recommended in the treatment of osteoarthritis in dogs.

As with all supplements, you should make sure that the product you choose is of good quality and is properly formulated. The most important things to look for in selecting an omega-3 fatty acid supplement are the ratio of omega-3 to omega-6, the amount (concentration) and the quality. Work with your veterinarian to find a high-quality dog food designed for dogs with joint problems that meets all of your dog's needs, or find a high-quality omega-3 fatty acid supplement. Appendix E lists some "joint management" diets.

### Are There Any Disadvantages to the Use of Omega-3 Fatty Acids?

According to reports, fatty acid supplements rarely cause gastrointestinal problems, although sometimes dog owners claim that the supplement gives their dog "fish breath." Otherwise, the use of omega-3 fatty acids appears to be quite safe.

# What Is Glucosamine?

Glucosamine is a kind of sugar that is found in large quantities in cartilage. Glucosamine was originally used as a supplement in the hope that it would encourage new cartilage to form. Glucosamine may work as an anti-inflammatory, which may help limit further cartilage destruction and pain and provide some benefits in the process of cartilage healing.

Glucosamine is derived from chitin, which is found in the shells of shellfish such as the Alaskan king crab. It is inexpensive and is found in many supplements. The purity of glucosamine may vary, depending on the way it is processed. Make sure to buy a highly purified product; less pure glucosamine supplements may contain contaminants or may even include substances that can cause an allergic reaction in your dog.

## What Is Chondroitin Sulfate?

**Chondroitin sulfate** is a complex molecule found in cartilage and in some other parts of the body. As we discussed earlier, the flow of water into and out of cartilage is vital to its function, and chondroitin sulfate is the most important molecule in the control of water in cartilage.

As osteoarthritis gets worse, the type and amount of chondroitin sulfate in the joints change, and the cartilage can't regulate the flow of water. Chondroitin sulfate is sometimes taken as a nutritional supplement in the hope that it will restore the normal water-binding process of cartilage and help the cartilage heal.

Chondroitin sulfate also can protect existing cartilage by blocking the actions of certain enzymes that lead to

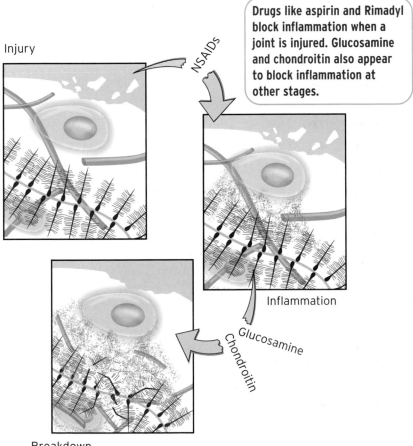

Injury

NSAIDs

Drugs like aspirin and Rimadyl block inflammation when a joint is injured. Glucosamine and chondroitin also appear to block inflammation at other stages.

Inflammation

Glucosamine
Chondroitin

Breakdown

breakdown in the joints. Chondroitin sulfate has been shown in the laboratory to improve healing of cartilage, but in real-life situations this ability still seems uncertain.

Chondroitin sulfate has been shown to have major anti-inflammatory effects. In combination with glucosamine, it may decrease the need for NSAIDs. A specific combination of chondroitin sulfate and high-purity glucosamine has been shown to slow down cartilage damage better than using either of these compounds alone. Chondroitin sulfate comes from many sources, including shark cartilage and the cartilage of cows and pigs.

Chondroitin sulfate supplements differ quite a bit in terms of cost and quality. The amount and quality of chondroitin sulfate in nutritional supplements are a big concern. One university study of human nutritional supplements showed that some products had less than 10% of the chondroitin sulfate that was listed on the label. Overall, just 16% of the products studied met the claims found on their labels. Another study of veterinary products found just one glucosamine/chondroitin sulfate product that met the claims on its label. When selecting a product, choose carefully (see p. 106). The Food and Drug Administration (FDA) has posted a list of guidelines for choosing a quality supplement on its Web site (www.cfsan.gov/~dms/ds-savvy.html). Important considerations include the following:

- **What information does the manufacturer have to prove the claims made for the product? Keep in mind that sometimes manufacturers supply so-called proof of their claims by showing undocumented reports from satisfied consumers or internal graphs and charts that could be mistaken for quality research.**
- **Does the manufacturer have information to share about tests it has conducted on the safety or usefulness of the ingredients in the product?**
- **Does the manufacturer have a quality-control system in place to show whether the product actually contains what is stated on the label and that the product is free of contaminants?**
- **Has the manufacturer received any reports of adverse events from consumers using the product?**

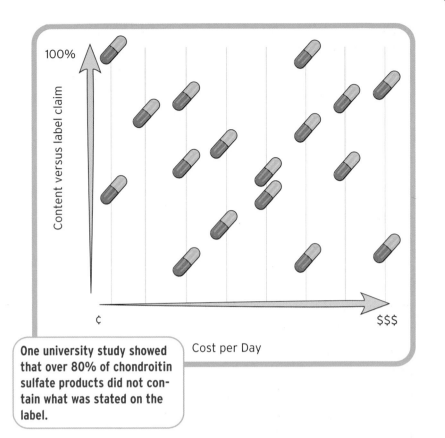

100%

Content versus label claim

¢                                        $$$

Cost per Day

One university study showed that over 80% of chondroitin sulfate products did not contain what was stated on the label.

## How Does Vitamin C Work?

Vitamin C helps build new cartilage by producing **collagen,** a tough, ropy protein that's found in cartilage. Vitamin C also is considered an antioxidant, and it may help ease inflammation. It's often found in combination products with glucosamine and chondroitin sulfate.

## What about MSM?

MSM, short for methylsulfonylmethane, is derived from DMSO, or dimethylsulfoxide. DMSO is a byproduct of wood pulp processing and is available as both industrial-grade and pharmaceutical-grade products. The pharmaceutical-grade product is approved in the United States only as a treatment for interstitial cystitis, a urinary tract disorder, in people. DMSO has a strong odor and taste, so MSM, which does not have these unpleasant characteristics, was developed as an alternative. MSM is said to have the anti-inflammatory effects of pharmaceutical-grade

DMSO, but most support for MSM is based on anecdotal (non-scientific) reports. A few studies have been conducted, but only in laboratory animals. There have been no studies of the effectiveness or safety of MSM in dogs. Safety is a concern because the MSM on the market comes from the industrial-grade form, and not from the pharmaceutical-grade DMSO.

## What about Perna Mussel?

Manufacturers of supplements containing Perna mussel, also known as the green-lipped mussel, claim that these products help alleviate the symptoms of osteoarthritis. In some human scientific studies, Perna mussel has been shown to ease the inflammation of **rheumatoid arthritis** and osteoarthritis of the **stifle.** Perna mussel has not, however, been definitively shown in controlled scientific studies to have any beneficial effects on osteoarthritis and cartilage repair in dogs. One study showed that giving Perna mussel to dogs did not result in significant improvement in the dogs' mobility.

## What about Other Supplements?

Many other supplements have been recommended for the treatment of osteoarthritis in people and dogs, including creatine, yucca, and Boswellia.

At this time there just is not enough scientific information to justify the use of these supplements, and there has not been enough testing to determine their safety. For these reasons, their use in the treatment of osteoarthritis is not generally recommended.

# How Much Should I Give?

Unfortunately, there is not much scientific information on the proper dosages of nutritional supplements. Dosage recommendations vary, depending on the manufacturer or the veterinarian. The dosages of supplements in dog foods are based mainly on the calorie needs of the dog. Because many dogs with osteoarthritis are overweight, you should be more concerned with helping your dog lose weight than with getting the "right amount" of supplement into the dog in the form of dog food.

There is very little clinical evidence regarding the use of supplements, so the dosages of these products are based mostly on anecdotal evidence.

We recommend the following approximate dosages:

| Body Weight | Glucos- amine | Chondroitin | Frequency |
|---|---|---|---|
| 10–24 lb | 500 mg | 400 mg | Once a day |
| 25–49 lb | 1000 mg | 800 mg | Once a day |
| 50–100 lb | 1000 mg | 800 mg | Once or twice a day |
| >100 lb | 1000 mg | 800 mg | Twice a day |

# Are There Any Risks?

The products in most nutritional supplements used to treat osteoarthritis in dogs are safe, especially omega-3 fatty acids, glucosamine, and chondroitin sulfate. From time to time an owner reports stomach upset in his or her dog when it has been given a nutritional supplement, although in most cases it isn't possible to establish a direct association between the supplement and the stomach upset.

The greatest risk of nutritional supplements is purchasing a product that is poorly manufactured. The end result is a waste of your money and a loss of any benefit your dog would have gotten from a better-made supplement.

# Who Regulates Nutritional Supplements?

At this time the government doesn't require testing and regulation of nutritional supplements. Independent testing has shown that not all labels can be trusted, even when the words "guaranteed analysis" appear.

Independent, voluntary laboratory testing of the quality of supplements is available, and there is also information on some products for dogs. One source for such information is ConsumerLab.com.

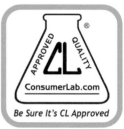

# How Do I Choose a Brand?

Before choosing a dog food made for dogs with osteoarthritis, talk to your veterinarian. The diet you choose should provide the appropriate supplements (generally omega-3 fatty acids) for osteoarthritis and supply the proper number of calories for weight management. All of

## Where We Stand

Nutritional supplements for the treatment of osteoarthritis are aggressively marketed and are often expensive. Even though most of these products are safe, the quality and content of these poorly regulated products are major concerns. We recommend that our patients with osteoarthritis be given high-quality supplements that have been tested by an independent laboratory.

the major therapeutic diets are well manufactured, and unlike many independent supplements, they accurately describe their contents on the label. In certain cases, particularly if your dog needs a therapeutic diet that doesn't contain omega-3 fatty acids, you can supplement the diet with a product such as Derm-caps or another omega-3 fatty acid product.

If you choose to buy a **nutraceutical** in addition to or instead of a joint diet, we recommend nutritional supple-

## Where We Stand

### Do Supplements Really Work?

Figuring out whether supplements really help dogs with osteoarthritis is not easy. The highest level of testing requires high-quality trials that are:

- Well designed
- Randomized
- Controlled

The best evidence relies on several components, including:

- Client questionnaires
- Veterinarians' evaluations
- Computerized lameness evaluations

Few products are ever subjected to this level of testing. Some of the therapeutic dog foods have been tested in this fashion, and the results are promising. Unfortunately, most dietary products for the treatment of osteoarthritis in dogs have not been and likely never will be tested. It's up to you to understand the importance of quality testing, and it's up to the veterinarian to help you make the most educated decision possible.

## Where We Stand

### Putting It All Together

The main goal of diet in the treatment of joint disease is achieving and maintaining the correct weight. The secondary goal is proper supplementation, most importantly with omega-3 fatty acids and glucosamine and chondroitin. Achieving both of these goals requires different diets in different dogs. In some cases it may be possible to use a commercially available diet that helps the dog maintain the proper weight while providing proper supplementation. In other cases a dog may need to be fed both a specialty dog food and individual supplements. In still other cases it may be necessary to change the dog food to achieve and then maintain the proper weight. You should always work with your veterinarian to achieve these goals and to make sure that your dog's diet is having the best possible effect on your dog's comfort and function.

ments that contain glucosamine *and* chondroitin sulfate, because combination therapy with these two ingredients has been shown to be more effective than either one alone. You may see manganese and vitamin C as additional ingredients in such products. We recommend only brands that have been tested for quality and content by an independent laboratory such as ConsumerLab.com. Ask your veterinarian for recommendations, and find out whether the product has been independently tested. Also, check the FDA's Web site for advice on choosing a quality supplement: www.cfsan.gov/~dms/ds-savvy.html. The FDA recommends choosing a supplement that has been documented safe and effective in published research.

# What about Cost?

Nutritional supplements vary tremendously in cost, but keep in mind that high cost doesn't guarantee high quality. The university study we mentioned earlier showed that even the more expensive chondroitin sulfate products did not always contain the amount of chondroitin sulfate listed on their labels. Again, before investing in an expensive product, make sure that it has been independently tested.

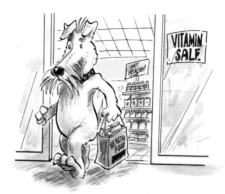

Now let's review the information in this chapter:

- **Most nutritional supplements are intended to treat osteoarthritis by easing inflammation and pain.**
- **Nutritional supplements have not been shown to help greatly in healing osteoarthritis.**
- **The most important nutritional supplements for dogs with osteoarthritis are fatty acids, glucosamine, and chondroitin.**
- **Omega-3 fatty acids (also known as DHA, EPA, and fish oil) are best provided in foods made especially for dogs with osteoarthritis.**
- **Omega-3 fatty acids have been shown to ease the pain and inflammation of osteoarthritis in dogs.**
- **Many glucosamine and chondroitin products do not contain what their labels claim.**
- **There is conflicting evidence that glucosamine and chondroitin supplementation ease the pain and inflammation of osteoarthritis in dogs.**
- **There is no significant evidence that other nutritional supplements help treat osteoarthritis in dogs.**

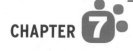

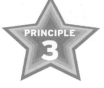

# Appropriate Exercise

**Osteoarthritis can be made worse if your dog gets too much or too little exercise. The right type and amount of exercise can provide excellent benefits to dogs with osteoarthritis. In this chapter we explore how exercise affects osteoarthritis and what kinds of exercise (and how much) are best for your dog.**

# Exercise and Osteoarthritis

The third principle of management of osteoarthritis is modification and moderation of exercise. Too much or too little exercise can make osteoarthritis worse, but the right kind and amount of exercise can provide great benefits to a dog with osteoarthritis. In this chapter we'll explain how exercise affects osteoarthritis and talk about which kinds of exercise (and how much of them) are best for your dog.

Research in people shows that exercise is one of the best treatments for osteoarthritis. Exercise improves mood and outlook, decreases pain, increases flexibility, improves the heart and blood flow, maintains weight, and promotes general physical fitness. The same is true of dogs. We all know that dogs love activity, but osteoarthritis can limit a dog's ability to exercise. In fact, one of the most common signs of osteoarthritis is **exercise intolerance**—the dog can't exercise for as long or as hard as she has in the past. Often a dog shows signs of exercise intolerance long before the owner notices any specific limping. Family members must learn to recognize the signs that a pet is exercising too hard or too fast and know when to stop or slow down to prevent pain and injury.

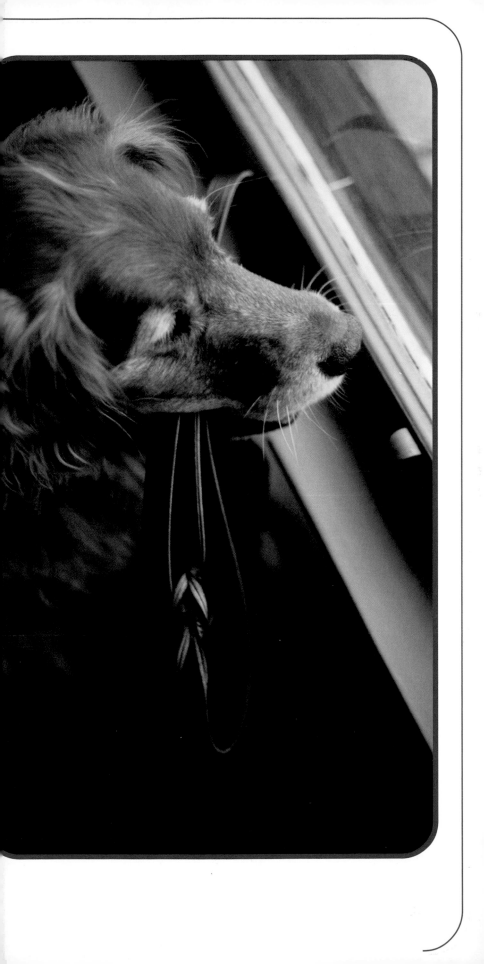

# Can Exercise Cause Osteoarthritis?

Normal joints in people—and dogs—of all ages tolerate long periods of hard exercise without bad effects or faster development of osteoarthritis, so normal exercise doesn't cause osteoarthritis. Exercise may actually help prevent osteoarthritis by making the muscles around the joint stronger and helping the joint become more stable and flexible. Overexercise can make the signs and pain of osteoarthritis worse, though, especially in overweight patients.

# How Does Exercise Help in the Treatment of Osteoarthritis?

Exercise helps dogs with osteoarthritis in many ways. The most important benefits are helping the dog lose weight, strengthening the muscles, and improving range of motion of the joints.

## Exercise and Weight Loss

The first principle of management of osteoarthritis is losing excess weight and keeping the weight at a healthy level. As outlined in Chapter 5, weight control is achieved through a combination of diet changes and proper exercise. The right kind of exercise helps a dog lose weight by getting rid of fat and increasing the amount of muscle the dog carries on its body.

Unfortunately, it can be difficult and painful for a dog with severe osteoarthritis to exercise, especially if the dog is obese. If your dog is obese and has **arthritis** bad enough to keep him from exercising, you'll have to work closely with your veterinarian to change your dog's diet

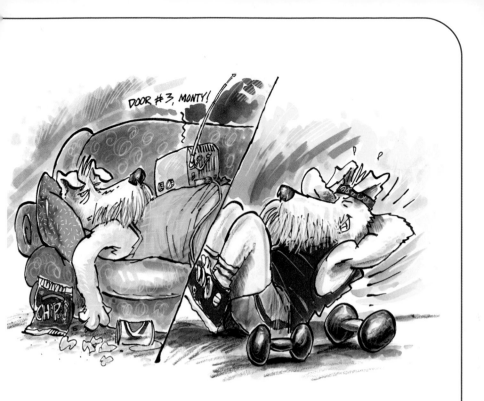

Research shows that people with osteoarthritis who take part in their own care report less pain and make fewer doctor visits. For the same reasons, every member of the family should take part in caring for the dog.

and increase the exercise your dog gets to help him lose weight and get around easier.

Your dog doesn't have to exercise hard to lose weight. Just as in people, slow walking benefits weight reduction. If your dog doesn't want to go even on short walks, you and your veterinarian should come up with a plan, including a low-calorie diet and anti-inflammatory medication, to relieve your dog's pain so that she can begin some mild exercise.

## The PPET Program: People and Pets Exercising Together

Recently Northwestern Memorial Hospital teamed with Hill's Pet Nutrition to study the benefits people and their pets get from exercising together. In this study of about 100 overweight people, approximately half were asked to follow an exercise program that included their dogs; the other half exercised without a pet. The results showed benefits for both the people and their pets. The combined dog/owner weight-loss program was better at keeping the people (and their dogs) in regular exercise. The authors of the study concluded that companion dogs can serve as social support for human weight loss and maintenance and that the people in the pet exercise group were getting more physical activity by taking part in dog-related activities. The people who exercised with their pets also reported much better quality of life. The dogs benefited from increased regular exercise and their owners' involvement in weight loss.

A similar study has been completed by the Bassett Healthcare Center in cooperation with the Iams Company. The results were similar. The researchers found health benefits for both the owners and the pets involved in the program.

The results of these studies support the belief that exercising with your pet can have social and medical benefits for both of you. Getting into the habit of exercising with your dog can help both of you through improved weight management, increased exercise, and improved quality of life.

For more information on the PPET program, visit www.petfit.com/Petfit/PetIndex.jsp.

## Exercise and Muscle Strengthening

One of the most important things exercise does for dogs with osteoarthritis is to make the muscles stronger. A dog with osteoarthritis experiences pain, causing the dog to stop moving around as much as before and to use the painful leg as little as possible. This lack of exercise causes the loss of muscle mass, or **atrophy**, all over the body and in the painful leg in particular. Muscle is one of the major support structures that keep joints from moving abnormally and being damaged. Of the four major stabilizing structures—muscle, joint shape, joint capsule, and **ligaments**—only muscle can easily be made stronger. An unstable joint puts the dog at risk for cartilage damage, soft tissue injury around the joint, and pain. (Think back to when you've twisted your ankle or had a similar injury.) Making the muscles around a joint stronger prevents the joint from moving in the wrong way and eases the pain. Exercise is the best way to make the muscles stronger.

## Exercise and Range of Motion

As we've just discussed, exercise can strengthen the muscles around a joint to make them more stable. At the same time, it increases your dog's ability to move the joint normally. The normal variation in movement of a joint is referred to as its **range of motion**. Osteoarthritis causes a buildup of scar tissue in the soft tissues around

### Structures That Keep Joints Stable

- Bones
- Joint capsules
- Ligaments
- Muscles

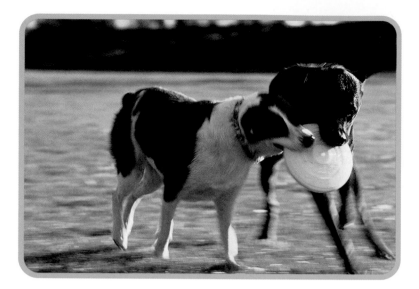

a joint, limiting the range of motion. You may see this in your dog as a stiffness and inability to do normal activities such as jumping into a car or climbing the stairs.

Careful exercise can dramatically improve joint range of motion in your dog by slowly stretching the scar tissue around the joint. This stretching, combined with muscle strengthening, can help your dog get back the ability to do normal activities.

## Exercise and Quality of Life

We all know that dogs love to run and play. Osteoarthritis and excess weight can really limit a dog's ability to take part in these activities. By helping your dog lose weight and exercise more, you can improve your dog's health, probably extend its lifespan, and improve your dog's quality of life.

# Can Exercise Make Osteoarthritis Worse?

Uncontrolled exercise—too hard or too fast—can hurt a joint, just as carefully controlled exercise—the right kind of exercise in the right amounts—can make joints healthier. Exercising too much or too hard can harm a joint by damaging soft tissues and cartilage.

# Damage to Soft Tissues

Osteoarthritis leads to **fibrosis**, or formation of scar tissue, around the affected joints. Scar tissue isn't very flexible, so the range of motion in an arthritic joint is less than that of a normal joint. A dog that suddenly becomes more active may move its joints in a way that causes the joint capsule to stretch or tear, and the dog will experience pain and limping. Exercise should be controlled so that the joint capsule is stretched slowly over time, without causing much pain. Try to avoid activities and play involving movements such as jumping and twisting until the joint has been stretched properly and these movements no longer cause your dog serious pain.

# Contribution to Cartilage Wear

Excessive exercise or intense movement can contribute to cartilage damage in several ways. In a joint with **dysplasia,** too much activity can make cartilage wear away faster by causing grinding of unhealthy cartilage surfaces. In an unstable joint, certain activities can help make carti-

## Where We Stand

Some of the activities that you may enjoy most with your dog, including playing fetch, playing chase, and roughhousing, can cause pain in the arthritic dog and make the osteoarthritis get worse faster. As orthopedic surgeons, we are concerned most with your dog's quality of life, so we're not telling you to cut out these activities entirely. Instead, try moderating these activities and avoid the ones that can cause irreparable harm to the joints. We also strongly recommend that you give your dog anti-inflammatory medication before any vigorous activity; this is most effective in limiting your dog's pain.

lage wear away by causing your dog to move the joint in the wrong way. In an arthritic joint, the wrong kind or wrong intensity of exercise stresses fragile cartilage and speeds up the wear and tear on the joint.

# Achieving a Balance

Many of the same activities that you and your dog love—playing fetch, chasing, wrestling with other dogs—make arthritis worse. We're not telling you to eliminate these activities from your dog's life, but do keep in mind that these activities may cause pain and may make arthritis get worse faster. The best thing to do is to moderate the amount of these activities, to keep pain to a minimum and avoid significant injury that can't be reversed. Try to anticipate when your dog will be especially active and give the dog anti-inflammatory medications before the fun starts.

# Controlled Voluntary Exercise

Exercise is divided clinically into four groups: passive, active assisted, active resistive, and controlled voluntary. We'll talk about the first three types in Chapter 8, which is about physical rehabilitation. In this chapter we'll focus on the most common kind: controlled voluntary exercise.

Most human and veterinary orthopedic surgeons and physical therapists agree that a good activity for arthritic joints helps make muscles stronger and improves the range of motion while avoiding heavy impact on the joint. For this reason, the best activities are swimming and controlled walking.

## Swimming

Swimming may be the single best activity for arthritic joints. We and our dogs are buoyant in water (we both float), easing the impact of exercise on cartilage, while

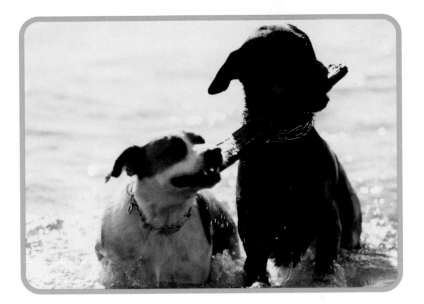

the motions of swimming require the swimmer to use full motion of the joints. Swimming helps increase flexibility and strength, making it a perfect activity for a dog with osteoarthritis.

Keep a few precautions in mind when you take your dog swimming. Make sure that the places where your dog will get in and out of the water are safe. Your dog may need help getting into a pool, and you should try to keep her from running into and out of natural bodies of water with rocky shores. The water temperature should not be so low that it makes your dog's arthritis discomfort worse. Finally, don't allow your dog to swim for so long that she gets overtired or exhausted.

## Walking

Controlled walking is another excellent activity for arthritic dogs. On a soft surface such as grass, it's fairly gentle on cartilage. You can help your dog increase range of motion of the joints by having your dog walk in high weeds. Walking slowly up hills will help your dog build muscle strength.

When you take your dog for a walk, look for soft surfaces whenever you can, and keep the walk short enough for your dog to remain comfortable .

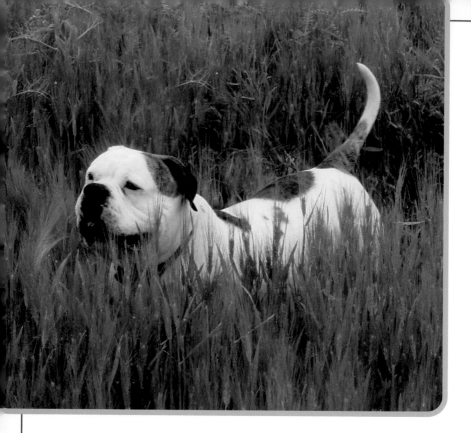

## Running and Playing

Running and playing are uncontrolled voluntary exercise. Running, especially on hard surfaces, is a high-impact activity. It helps your dog build endurance and is a great way to burn calories, but it doesn't help your dog become flexible and gain muscle strength like other exercises do. It's best to take your dog running on soft surfaces. Don't take your pet distance running until you've checked with your veterinarian or veterinary rehabilitation therapist.

Play, such as fetching, chasing, jumping, and wrestling with other dogs, often involves sudden turns and twists that can stretch or tear the scar tissue around arthritic joints. A dog with arthritis is often limping after these activities, so keep an eye on your dog and limit this sort of activity, depending on the kind of injury and how severe it is.

# How Much Exercise and When?

In starting an exercise program for your pet, you and other family members should adopt a healthy outlook. You'll see the best results when you and your family work together to accomplish the goals you've set with the help of your veterinarian (and veterinary rehabilitation therapist, when available). People with osteoarthritis who take part in their own care report less pain and visit their doctors less often, and this probably is true for dogs as well.

The kind and amount of exercise a dog with joint disease should get depend on several factors, including the dog's weight and overall health, recent surgery or trauma, and the type of injury.

# Exercise after Surgery

When your dog has surgery, you must follow the discharge instructions of your veterinary surgeon closely. Not following directions can have disastrous results, including the need for costly new surgeries and even the loss of limb function. Never increase your dog's activity level or start a new kind of exercise until you've checked with your veterinary surgeon.

Exercise after surgery is almost always limited so that your dog's soft tissues, cartilage, and bone have a chance to heal. Your surgeon may not let you increase your dog's activity or start any significant exercise until he or she has examined the dog and can see that the dog has healed enough. How much you'll have to limit your dog's activity and how long you'll have to do it will depend on many factors, including the dog's age, the kind of injury that was repaired by the surgeon, and how severe the injury was. Younger animals heal much faster, but they're more likely to form scar tissue that can limit the flexibility of a joint or limb. Older animals may take much longer to heal, especially when bone is involved. Bone heals slowly, and your veterinarian will check your dog's progress using x-rays. When bone is injured, it's best to limit your dog's movement so that the bone can heal—but this same limitation makes it possible for restrictive scar tissue to form. Cartilage doesn't heal well, but any healing that does take place usually occurs during the 4 weeks after trauma or surgery. Cartilage heals best when the joint stays in motion but your dog doesn't put as much weight on the injury. For these reasons, your veterinarian will decide the proper timing and type of rehabilitation after carefully considering the structures involved, plus other factors such as the age of your dog. See Chapter 10 for typical discharge instructions for a dog that's undergone a common orthopedic surgical procedure.

# Professional Exercise Programs

Professional exercise programs are usually designed by a veterinary rehabilitation therapist for a particular dog with a specific injury. The program may include regular appointments with the rehabilitation therapist, activities for you and your dog to do at home, or both. If money, time, or distance keeps you from having regular visits with a veterinary rehabilitation therapist, think about making just a few visits to design a program and evaluate your dog's progress. These programs are designed to control weight, ease pain, and improve function. Ask your veterinarian for a referral to a qualified rehabilitation therapist if you are interested in setting up an individualized exercise program for your dog.

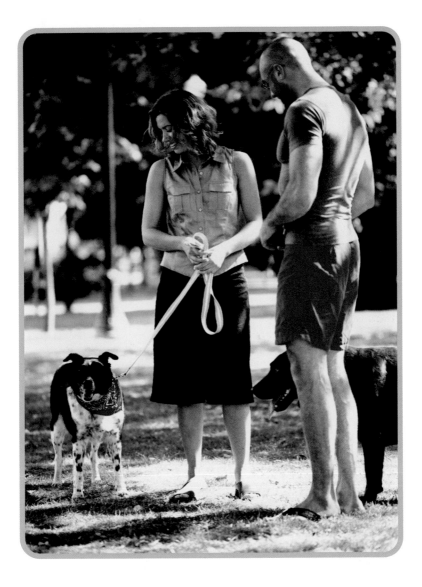

# Exercise for Overweight Dogs with Joint Disease

A dog that's very overweight may not be used to exercise and may have other medical problems, too. If your dog has not gotten much exercise for a long time, check with your veterinarian before starting any vigorous exercise. Remember, even mild exercise can help your overweight dog lose weight and improve function. Often, an

## Where We Stand

### Exercise for the Overweight Dog with Joint Disease

In many cases, an overweight dog with serious joint disease, especially osteoarthritis, doesn't want to exercise because it hurts. If this is the case with your dog, work with your veterinarian to come up with a program that combines a weight-loss diet, pain medications, and exercise for a change to a healthier lifestyle.

overweight dog with severe joint disease, especially osteoarthritis, doesn't want to exercise because it hurts. In such a case, the dog's owner should work with the veterinarian to come up with a program that combines a weight-loss diet, pain medications, and exercise to help the dog live a healthier lifestyle.

Start slowly. We recommend the controlled exercise of walking your dog on a leash. Encourage your dog, but don't make the dog walk until he can't go any farther. Try to exercise an hour or so after giving your dog the anti-inflammatory drug your veterinarian has prescribed. This will give your dog the greatest pain relief during the exercise. Start with walks of 5 to 10 minutes on a flat surface, adding 5 to 10 minutes each week. Once you and your dog are up to 30 or 40 minutes, think about starting more vigorous exercise, such as walking on hills or swimming. Be sure that your dog is healthy and that the water is warm enough before starting swimming exercises.

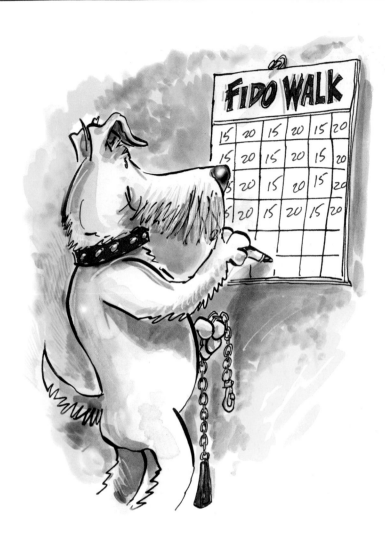

# Exercise for Healthy Dogs with Joint Disease

Owners of dogs with osteoarthritis should develop daily routines to promote healthy exercise. Changing activities every so often will help prevent boredom and keep your dog enthusiastic about exercising.

Regular physical activity and rest are important in keeping your dog healthy. In the same way, it's important

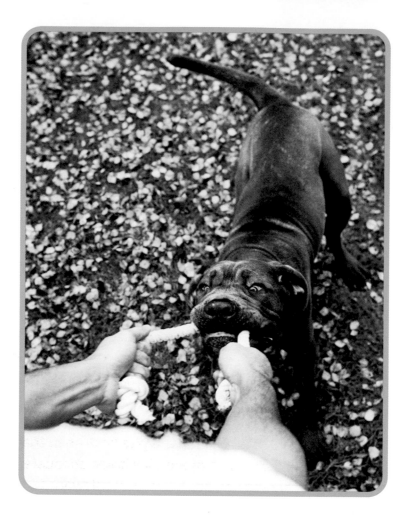

to avoid injury caused by overuse. **Episodic activity**—activity that the animal does for a reasonable period several times a day, with rest in between—is usually best for the treatment of osteoarthritis. Leading a couch-potato life during the week and exercising hard only on the weekend can actually make osteoarthritis worse instead of improving your dog's function and quality of life. In addition to making the osteoarthritis worse, this approach is very likely to cause serious injury. Every treatment plan should include regularly scheduled rest.

# Advanced Exercise Therapy

Two types of exercise are important in treating osteoarthritis. The first kind, therapeutic exercise, keeps joints working as well as they can. Therapeutic exercise calls for low-impact activity, and specific exercises are designed to maintain or increase range of motion, reflexes, and elasticity of soft tissues. Massage, water therapy, and activities in which you or someone else moves or stretches your dog's joints are all examples of therapeutic exercise. (These techniques are discussed in detail in Chapter 8.) The other type of exercise, aerobic conditioning, improves strength and fitness and controls weight. Brisk walking, walking or trotting through high grass, and swimming are all examples of aerobic exercise.

## Warmup

Most dogs with osteoarthritis exercise best when their pain is less severe. Start your dog off with an adequate warmup and have the dog begin exercising slowly. Frequent breaks will help him get a good workout but keep the risk of overuse injury low. As a warmup, you might walk your dog slowly, put a warm pack over the site of injury, massage your dog gently, move his joints in the range in which it's comfortable, or give your pet a session of warm-water massage. Any combination of these activities enjoyed by your pet will serve as a good warmup for the exercise period.

One osteoarthritis study in human beings showed that the people who had kept most closely to their exercise regimens were the ones with the lowest levels of disability at the end of the study. The same is probably true of dogs.

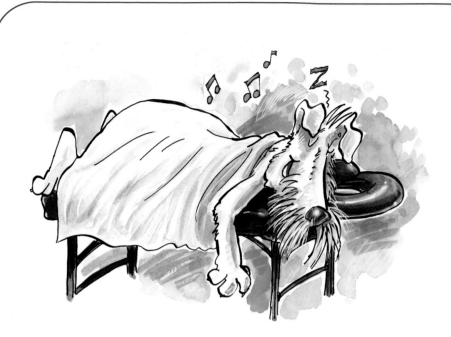

## Strength and Endurance

A well-designed exercise and rehabilitation plan includes activities that will strengthen your dog's muscles, plus help build its endurance, range of motion, flexibility, and balance.

In strengthening exercises, the muscles are required to carry a high load for a limited number of contractions. The diameter and number of muscle fibers increase in response to this exercise, and as a result, the target muscle gets bigger. Stair-climbing, "down-to-stand" exercises, and "sit-to-stand" exercises are all examples of strength exercises. Endurance activities involve lighter loads but higher numbers of contractions. Aquatic treadmill therapy and long walks are both examples of endurance exercises. Range-of-motion activities increase the elasticity of soft tissues. Walking through high grass, aquatic treadmill therapy, Cavelletti jumping, and incline work are all range-of-motion activities. Balance activities improve your dog's reflexes and the brain's sense of where the muscles are and what they're doing, helping your dog avoid further injury. Physioroll activity (walking while supported by a large rubber ball) and balance-board activity are both examples of balance activities. Your veterinarian and veterinary rehabilitation therapist can evaluate your pet and come up with activities for your family to do with your pet at home.

## Cool Down

After exercise, it's important to have a cool-down period followed by rest. Your dog needs a period of real rest to allow the tissues to recover from exercise. During this time, help your dog relax and de-stress by offering petting and praise for the good work. Stress-relaxation techniques are helpful in people, and the same is probably true of our pets.

Now let's review the information in this chapter:

- **Normal exercise doesn't cause osteoarthritis, but too much exercise can make the signs and pain of osteoarthritis worse, particularly in an overweight dog.**
- **The right kind of exercise, in the right amounts, is good for a dog with osteoarthritis because it helps control weight, increases muscle strength, and improves the dog's range of motion.**
- **Exercise can do wonders for a dog's attitude and quality of life.**
- **Swimming and walking, called "controlled voluntary exercises," are some of the best activities you can do with your dog.**
- **After surgery, your veterinarian will give you guidelines for your dog's exercise, and it will be your job to follow them carefully.**

# Physical Rehabilitation

**PRINCIPLE 4**

In dogs, physical therapy is often called rehabilitation. Physical rehabilitation is the use of techniques that help restore function, improve mobility, relieve pain, and prevent or limit permanent physical disabilities in patients with injuries or disease. Even though rehabilitation is not needed or used in every case of arthritis, it has been found very effective in many cases of joint disease in dogs. Physical therapy and rehabilitation have long been used to help people recover from orthopedic surgery and to improve function and ease the pain of joint disease. Now, the benefits of rehabilitation are recognized in veterinary medicine, particularly for dogs with joint disease. It's just one part of a new specialty that includes canine sports medicine and canine physical rehabilitation.

## What Is Physical Rehabilitation?

Rehabilitation varies in scope quite a bit, from simple techniques using limited tools to advanced methods involving sophisticated equipment. Professional rehabilitation requires time and expense, but in many cases you may be able to apply simple methods of rehabilitation yourself once your veterinarian or rehabilitation therapist has shown you how. Advanced rehabilitation techniques will require the skill and equipment of a canine rehabilitation professional. Professional treatments are generally used in more complicated cases and often involve working and performance dogs, although more pet owners are also choosing professional physical rehabilitation for their dogs.

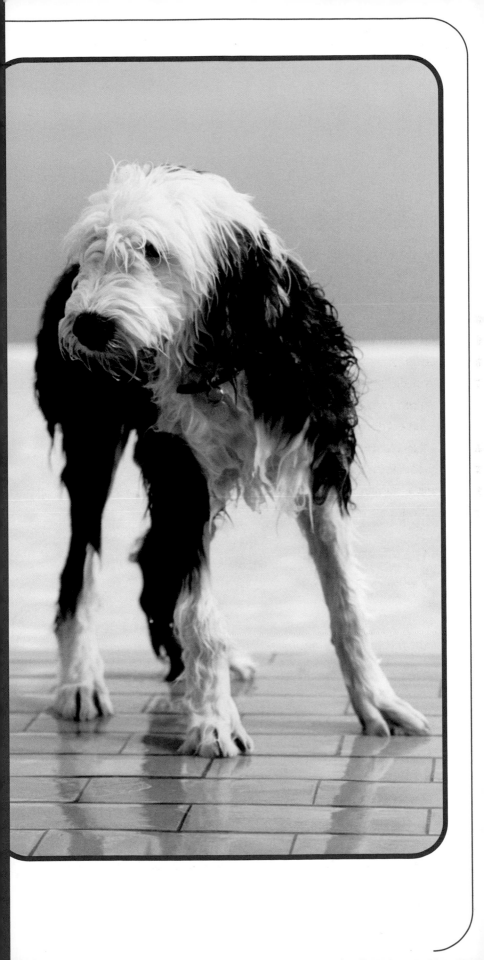

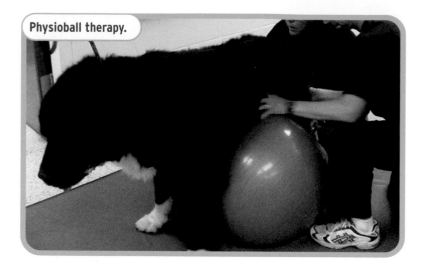

Physioball therapy.

In this chapter we'll discuss the function and forms of physical rehabilitation and help you understand which types of treatment should be applied and by whom.

# Do I Need a Professional Rehabilitation Therapist?

Rehabilitation may be carried out by a veterinarian, a trained veterinary rehabilitation therapist, or you, the dog's owner, once you are trained in the proper techniques. Deciding if you need a professional therapist should be based on your veterinarian's recommendation and on your personal goals and financial choices.

## Where We Stand

Rehabilitation should always be supervised by a veterinarian skilled in rehabilitation or a rehabilitation therapist because of the risk of injury.

# Who Is Qualified as a Professional Rehabilitation Therapist?

In choosing a rehabilitation professional, make sure to ask about the person's qualification or training.

Certification programs and continuing education programs provide training for veterinarians, veterinary technicians, physical rehabilitation therapists, and physical rehabilitation assistants.

The rehabilitation therapist coordinates and performs therapeutic treatments with the cooperation of the owner and the veterinarian. The American Veterinary Medical Association's guidelines state that all treatments must be conducted by or supervised by a veterinarian. This helps guarantee that all therapies are appropriate for the problem being treated.

Most rehabilitation facilities only take dogs that have been referred by their veterinarians. To find a rehabilitation therapist in your area, ask your veterinarian or veterinary surgeon.

# How Does Physical Rehabilitation Help?

## Three Target Areas of Rehabilitation

Rehabilitation is intended to enhance the quality of life and function for your dog by improving the bones, joints, and muscles. The three main target areas of rehabilitation are:

- **Strength**
- **Endurance**
- **Range of motion**

## Strength

Strength training helps the patient with arthritis by increasing the stability of the joints. A joint with stronger muscle support is better protected from the stresses that occur with activities such as running and jumping. The number of fibers in a muscle can never be increased, although muscle fibers are lost as a dog gets older. The muscle fibers may also become smaller with disuse, a process called **atrophy**. Atrophy may occur as a result of disease, injury, lack of use, or lack of nerve impulses. Strengthening exercises can increase the size of muscle fibers; the muscle gets bigger, but the actual number of fibers does not increase. Strengthening exercises are similar to the exercises a human bodybuilder does. (A relatively high weight is placed on the muscle, after which a low number of repetitions are performed.)

## Endurance

**Endurance** is defined as the amount of time between the beginning of physical activity and the time when the activity must stop because of exhaustion or fatigue. Improved endurance helps a dog with arthritis return to her normal level of exercise. Endurance exercises increase the aerobic capacity of the muscle, making the muscle more resistant to fatigue. These exercises take

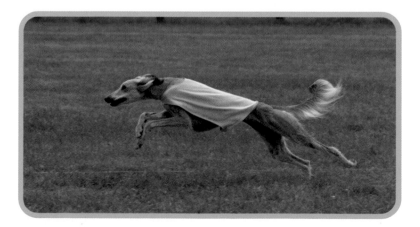

longer to do but put a low level of stress on the muscle; running and swimming are good examples.

## *Range of Motion*

Ideally, a dog's joints and limbs move freely and easily, without pain. The ability of a joint to move is called its **range of motion.** Arthritis causes a decrease in the range of motion because scar tissue forms around the joint and the muscles become more and more stiff, making it difficult for the dog to do activities such as climbing stairs or jumping up on a bed. Rehabilitation helps the dog regain the normal range of motion and return to full function, with less pain and stiffness.

Range of motion of a joint can be passive or active. Passive range of motion is the range of motion that is achieved when an outside force (such as a therapist) causes movement of a joint. It is usually the maximum range of motion that a joint can move. There may be some discomfort during passive range of motion.

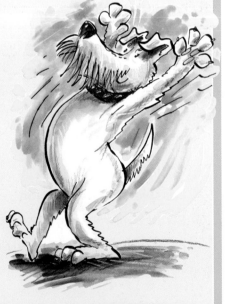

Active range of motion is the range of motion that the dog can achieve independently. Active range of motion is usually less than passive range of motion.

# Types of Rehabilitation

## Passive and Active Rehabilitation

Rehabilitation can be divided into two specific categories: passive (no active participation from the dog) and active (active participation by the dog). Passive treatments include cold and heat therapy, passive range-of-motion exercises (in which someone moves the dog's joints), stretching, massage therapy, electrical stimulation, and ultrasound. Active rehabilitation includes exercise therapy, **gait** training, and aquatic therapy.

### *Passive Rehabilitation Methods*

#### Thermal Agents

The application of heat or cold to raise or lower the temperature of the tissue around a joint can be used throughout a rehabilitation program. The choice of heat or cold depends on the tissue's stage of recovery.

## Typical Tools of Rehabilitation Therapy

### Passive

- **Cold/heat therapy**
- **Passive range of motion**
- **Stretching/massage therapy**
- **Electrical stimulation/ultrasound therapy**

### Active

- **Exercise therapy**
- **Gait training**
- **Aquatic therapy**

### How Cold Therapy Works

Superficial cold therapy reduces bleeding and swelling and decreases pain and muscle spasm. Cold therapy should be used following an injury or orthopedic surgery, or to treat muscular pain or soreness from exercising. In the management of arthritis, cold therapy is often applied immediately after surgery and up to several days thereafter. Your veterinarian may ask you to continue the cold therapy at home for several days to reduce the inflammation due to surgery and to make your dog feel better. Cold therapy can also be used by owners and trainers to aid in recovery after rehabilitation activities or exercises.

## How Cold Therapy Is Applied

Cold can be applied using ice packs, cold packs, or iced towels. In addition, compression can be applied with the cold to help reduce or prevent edema.

When applying cold treatments, place a thin layer of material between the cold pack and the dog's skin to increase the comfort level of your dog. Place a towel over the cold pack to avoid loss of cold to the environment. Cold therapy is usually applied for 20 minutes, once to four times a day. Even one application of cold during the first 24 hours of trauma has shown to be beneficial in the reduction of swelling and pain in human patients.

Cold should not be applied if the dog has cold hypersensitivity or decreased or absent sensation, and it should not be applied directly over areas with compromised circulation. The skin should be inspected if the dog shows unusual signs of discomfort.

### How Heat Therapy Works

Superficial heat therapy is used to increase metabolism, increase the flexibility of soft tissues, and decrease pain. Heat shouldn't be used until the signs of inflammation, such as heat, redness, and swelling, are gone. Heat is used to treat long-term traumatic and inflammatory conditions, muscle spasm, tissue tightness, and pain. In a dog with arthritis, heat may be used to help loosen tight muscles around a joint and improve their flexibility. Heat is often used several days or weeks after surgery, once inflammation has decreased.

## How Heat Therapy Is Applied

Superficial heat can be applied using heat packs, warm bath, shower massage, and whirlpools. Application time is 20 minutes two to four times per day. Inspect the skin at least every 5 minutes. Remove the heat source if your dog shows any signs of discomfort.

Heat therapy should not be used if any signs of inflammation are present, such as redness or swelling. Heat should not be used on dogs with decreased or absent sensation, over malignancies (cancer), or over an active infection.

### How Electrical Stimulation Works

Electrical stimulation can be used to increase muscle strength, to minimize muscle shrinking, for pain control, and to reduce the buildup of fluid. For safety's sake, only a trained rehabilitation therapist should use electrical stimulation. A dog's reaction to electrical stimulation may be unpredictable, and the therapist may recommend that your dog be muzzled to help keep her and the therapist safe.

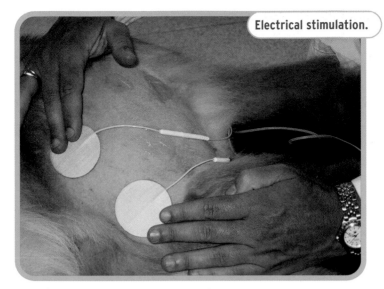

Electrical stimulation.

## How Therapeutic Ultrasound Works

In **therapeutic ultrasound,** an electric current is applied to a crystal, resulting in pressure waves that are absorbed by the tissues.

Therapeutic ultrasound can be used to increase blood flow, increase range of motion, decrease pain and muscle spasms, and speed up wound healing. Therapeutic ultrasound must be used with caution when a patient has been fitted with a plastic or metal-plate implant because the reflection of the pressure waves may cause more intense heating, leading to burns or discomfort.

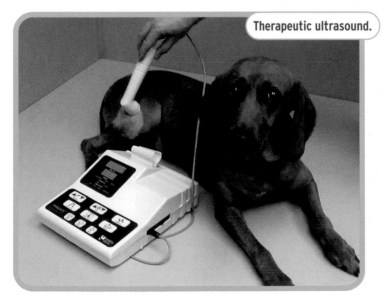

Therapeutic ultrasound.

## How Therapeutic Massage Works

Therapeutic massage, or the manipulation of soft tissue, improves function of the circulatory, muscular, skeletal, and nervous systems. It may help the body recover more quickly from injury or illness. Massage can be used to relax and reduce the anxiety of a dog recovering after surgery.

Two basic massage techniques are **effleurage** and **petrissage.** Effleurage is a gliding stroke that uses the whole hand. In petrissage, the person doing the massage uses a kneading compression stroke and rolls the dog's skin. It is used for muscle tension, knots, and spasms.

## How Passive Range-of-Motion Exercises Work

In passive range-of-motion exercises, the person giving the therapy moves the joint through as much of its flexion and extension as possible without causing discomfort.

Passive range of motion may be the most important exercise for a dog recovering from a joint injury or disease because it provides controlled motion without stressing the joint. To be beneficial, passive range of motion must be performed properly. Dog owners should review the range-of-motion techniques **very** carefully with their vet-

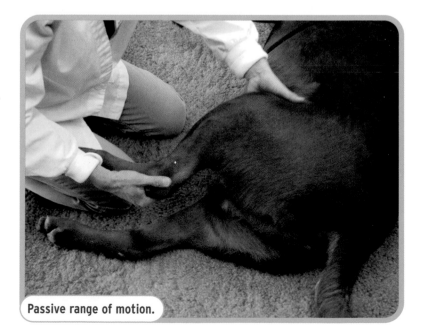

Passive range of motion.

erinarian or rehabilitation therapist before performing passive range of motion on their dog.

## Active Rehabilitation

### How Aquatic Therapy Works

In aquatic therapy, exercises are done in the water to help the dog gain strength, range of motion, and endurance while reducing the risk of injury. In the water a dog is able to contract its muscles without having to bear weight on them.

Aquatic therapy is excellent for soft tissue injuries, arthritis, muscle weakness, and overall conditioning. It should not be used for dogs with heart or lung disease, skin infections, or diarrhea.

The therapeutic properties of water include:

- Thermal
- Buoyancy
- Hydrostatic pressure
- Cohesion
- Turbulence

## Effect of Water Level on Body Weight

When the water level in a therapy tank is raised to the level of a dog's ankle, it reduces weight bearing by 9%. Basically the dog becomes 9% lighter on its feet and lower joints. The remaining 91% of the body weight is distributed by 40% in the rear limbs and 60% in the front limbs. The water level raised to the knee reduces the body weight by 15%. The water level raised to the hip reduces the body weight by 62%. The remaining 48% of the body weight is distributed by 29% in the rear limbs and 71% in the front limbs. This effect permits the rehabilitation therapist to accurately control the forces going through a dog's joints.

### Thermal Effects
The soothing effects of warm water ease pain and may help a dog exert more effort.

### Buoyancy
Exercises are done in the water to increase or decrease the amount of weight the dog must bear on its joints and bones. The actual effect of buoyancy can be very dramatic; reducing the body weight of the dog by even 10% can reduce the amount of stress on a weak joint and allow the dog to exercise more naturally and move more comfortably. The dog can move the joints without having to bear much weight on them, which is a huge help in rehabilitating diseased joints and limbs.

### Hydrostatic Effects
Hydrostatic pressure from water helps decrease swelling and promotes the normal flow of fluids through the limbs.

### Water Resistance
Cohesion and turbulence contribute to the resistance the dog encounters while moving through the water. The increased resistance helps improve muscle strength and endurance, helping the dog regain its previous athletic ability.

### Aquatic Therapy and the Underwater Treadmill
The **underwater treadmill** has rapidly become the most popular tool in the professional rehabilitation of dogs with musculoskeletal and other diseases. Many therapists and orthopedic surgeons consider exercise on this device better than swimming as a means of rehabilitation.

A therapist using the underwater treadmill can vary the water depth to increase or decrease the amount of weight the dog bears on the joints, can vary the speed of exercise, and can closely control the water temperature. On the other hand, underwater treadmills are available only through rehabilitation professionals and veterinarians, and their use requires training and strict supervision.

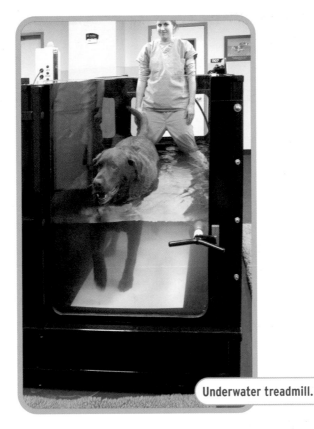

**Underwater treadmill.**

Swimming, which is an excellent exercise for the heart and blood vessels, is recommended when a dog shouldn't bear weight on the joints while exercising. Swimming is not as effective as the underwater treadmill in improving a dog's range of motion because it limits the extension of the joints—dogs tend to swim with their legs more flexed than they do while walking. Vigorous swimming can lead to muscle soreness and increased joint pain. On the plus side, swimming doesn't require expensive equipment, and sometimes, you, rather than a rehabilitation therapist, can supervise your dog as it swims.

### How Canine Exercise Therapy Works

Canine exercise therapy is an active rehabilitation technique involving the dog's natural ability to perform activities. It's designed to return the dog to function sooner and to lower the risk of injury in the future. The level of exercise varies with the condition of the dog or how long it has been since the dog had surgery.

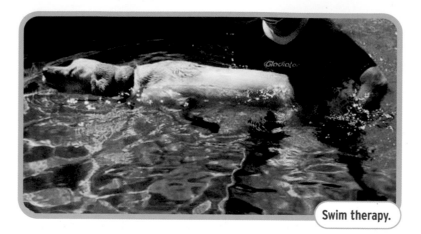

Swim therapy.

An exercise therapy program begins with short periods of low-impact activities and progresses to longer periods of more strenuous activities. You and your veterinarian or rehabilitation therapist should modify the program to accommodate your dog's comfort level. Remember, "comfort level" is different from "tolerance level": Your dog may continue a painful activity if you ask her to.

The exercise therapy program is divided into three stages: warmup, exercise activities, and postexercise therapy.

*Warmup* includes checking the dog's physical and mental condition and getting ready for the exercise session. You might prepare your dog for exercise by warming the painful area with a warm pack, shower massage, passive range-of-motion exercises, or stretching. Combining superficial heat and stretching is a great way to help your dog get the most from the exercise session.

The *exercise activities* usually include at least one exercise to increase strength, such as sit to stand; at least one exercise to increase endurance, such as walking; exercises to improve balance, such as use of a balance board or **physioball;** and at least one to improve or maintain range of motion, such as use of **Cavalletti poles** or walking in tall grass.

The cool-down portion of the program, or *postexercise therapy,* can include slow walking after vigorous exercise and application of ice to a previously injured area, to reduce any inflammation from microtrauma caused by exercise.

Often you can supervise your dog's exercise therapy at home. It is helpful, though, to meet with a rehabilitation therapist to get help in designing a program and to assess progress.

### How Gait Training Works

Chronic pain or traumatic injury can cause a dog to alter the way he walks or runs, known as the gait. Such a change can cause pain in or injury of nonarthritic legs. Gait training is intended to help the dog move as normally as possible.

# The Rehabilitation Program

As you now know, rehabilitation therapy for a dog with joint disease may involve the dog owner, a rehabilitation therapist, or both. Always consult your veterinarian before starting any rehabilitation program, especially if your dog has recently undergone surgery or has any medical conditions. Your veterinarian or rehabilitation therapist can help you design a program that meets both your dog's needs and your time and financial requirements.

The rehabilitation program begins with the evaluation of the dog. Each case is different, and you, the owner, are the key source of the information needed for your dog to have the best outcome possible.

## Evaluation

The evaluation is a combination of subjective and objective information. **Subjective information** is data provided by the owner; **objective information** is data collected during the examination. Both are important in figuring out the current condition of the dog.

### Subjective Information

The information you give your veterinarian or rehabilitation therapist—for example, age, breed, general appearance and disposition of the dog, details about the injury, and any pertinent medical history—is vital. The veterinarian or the rehabilitation therapist will ask you about your dog's home (and work) environment to find out whether your dog needs to be able to climb stairs or walk on slick floors. Whether you have other pets, especially other dogs, is also important because in the early part of rehabilitation you may have to keep your dog out of activities with other dogs to reduce the risk of injury. Knowing a dog's usual activity level helps the therapist figure out your dog's condition and will help you get a good understanding of what he should be able to do after rehabilitation. Knowing which medications and supplements your dog is taking and whether you believe they are helping can help the therapist assess the benefits of rehabilitation.

### Objective Evaluation

An objective evaluation gives your veterinary surgeon or rehabilitation therapist a starting point and knowledge of your dog's current abilities. It also helps them set goals

## Questions That Help Design a Rehabilitation Program

- **Does the dog refuse to go on walks? Is the dog slower to get up than before?**
- **Has the dog stopped jumping onto the couch?**
- **Does the dog refuse to climb or go down stairs?**
- **Is the dog unable to get into the car unassisted?**

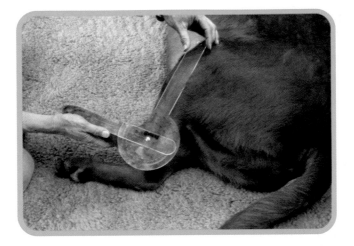

as a way of assessing progress. Several methods of evaluation may be used.

Passive range of motion is measured with a **goniometer,** an instrument like a protractor that measures the angle formed by two bones across a joint. The therapist will move the two bones to extreme flexion and extension and take a measurement at each point.

The therapist checks active range of motion by asking the dog to sit, stand, and lie down. The dog may also be asked to climb stairs or walk over poles.

The size of a muscle increases and decreases with the strength of the muscle. For this reason, the measurement around a front or rear leg muscle provides information about how much use or lack of use a dog has in one leg compared with the other.

"Body composition" is a term used to describe the ratio of body fat to lean muscle. It's measured by the therapist and recorded as a percentage.

## Gait Analysis

Gait analysis is the objective (using scientific measurement) or subjective (using the judgment of the observer) evaluation of how your dog moves whether walking or running or in any other activity. Abnormal gait or motion may be due to pain or dysfunction. Most of us perform gait analysis each day: We can see whether a person walking toward us is graceful or clumsy. We can tell whether a person who is running is balanced and fluid or stiff. The same observations apply to your dog.

The walk and trot are the easiest gaits to evaluate in a dog because of the symmetrical movement involved in them.

Subjective gait analysis is the tool used most often to diagnose **lameness.** It is best done before the therapist ever touches the dog. First the therapist watches the dog while she is still, looking for conformation abnormalities such as turned-out toes, or abnormalities in stance such as holding one leg up or putting most of the body weight on a particular leg. Next the therapist analyzes the dog while she is moving.

The dog's head movement, tail movement, stride length, symmetry, and front and rear movement are evaluated.

## Normal Gaits of the Dog

- **Walk—four-beat slow gait in which each foot lifts from the ground one at a time**

- **Amble—irregular four-beat gait that is faster than the walk; normal for Old English Sheep Dogs**

- **Pace—lateral two-beat gait; may be normal for some large breeds, but usually indicates a problem**

- **Trot—two-beat diagonal gait**

- **Flying trot—similar to trot, except faster, with more overreaching**

- **Canter—three-beat gait in which two legs move separately and two move as a pair**

- **Gallop—four-beat gait that looks like the canter, only faster, with a period of suspension**

Most gait analysis is qualitative or subjective, meaning that it is based on the assessment of the owner, veterinarian, or therapist. Objective gait analysis or scientifically measured analysis is performed using expensive and uncommon equipment called force platforms. This type of analysis is not routinely available and not necessary for routine rehabilitation.

## Determination of Goals

After assessment of the dog's condition is complete, rehabilitation goals and expectations are determined.

It is important to set reasonable goals at the beginning of the rehabilitation program. Thorough evaluation and assessment of the dog's current condition, your expectations as the dog's owner, and your commitment to the rehabilitation program provide information that's vital in developing the right program for your dog.

Expectations vary greatly, and you should be given the information and time to decide what your rehabilitation goals for your dog will be.

You and the therapist might set a goal for each phase of the rehabilitation. For example: in phase 1 (within 1 week), you might decide to set out to strengthen the back legs so that the dog can bear weight for at least 20 seconds without outside support. In phase 2, you might work on strengthening the dog's hind legs so that the dog can walk on the affected leg.

Rehabilitation goals keep the program focused, but they may change as your dog progresses.

## Designing the Rehabilitation Program

The rehabilitation program includes "methods" and "exercises." The methods include techniques such as cryotherapy, electrical stimulation, and ultrasound.

Exercises include walking, swimming, and other activities.

### Rehabilitation Methods

Many different types of methods and techniques can be used to reach the same rehabilitation goals. What works for one dog may not be right for another.

Therapies that should be performed by a trained rehabilitation therapist include therapeutic ultrasound, aquatic therapy, and electrical stimulation. The rehabilitation practitioner can develop a home exercise program to supplement the therapy your dog gets at the clinic and to maintain the strength, endurance, range of motion, and reflexes the dog has gained once rehabilitation has been completed.

### Rehabilitation Exercises

Exercises for the arthritic dog, which are low-impact, are done frequently. Most help the dog achieve pain-free movement by making the muscles around the affected area stronger and by increasing the dog's range of motion. It is important that you make sure your dog stays in her comfort zone during exercise.

Remember that rest is important during the exercise period, as well as throughout the day. A dog with arthritis requires rest periods during the exercise program for the cartilage to recover, for the muscles to rest, and for you to be sure that your dog is not sore after performing the exercises. A dog that is sore will tend to curl up and stay in one spot, putting the goals of the program at risk.

If a given exercise has made your dog sore, allow her to rest for a while; then have your dog walk for a few minutes every couple of hours to help keep her joints, **ligaments,** and muscle from tightening up.

### Exercise and the Older Dog

Special attention must be paid to older dogs. We recommend short, very-low-impact sessions of exercise. Most exercises for older dogs are focused on relaxation and range of motion.

# How Do You Know When Your Dog Has Achieved a Goal?

Outcome measurements help you be sure that rehabilitation goals are being met by showing how your dog is progressing as objectively as possible. Outcome measures are vital to providing the information needed to improve or change the rehabilitation program to ensure the most benefit for each dog. Documentation of the measurements provides progress information to you, the rehabilitation therapist, and the veterinarian.

# Home Physical Rehabilitation Techniques

This section includes examples of exercises that you can perform at home with your dog. Review these exercises with your veterinarian and have your dog evaluated to be sure that he is ready to begin an exercise program. Exercises in this section are divided into two categories: those that require no hands-on training for you and those that require you to be trained by the rehabilitation therapist to be effective and safe for your dog. Again, you can perform some of the exercises—those preceded by a green circle—at home with verbal instruction only. Others—those preceded by a yellow square—you should perform at home only after being trained by a rehabilitation practitioner.

## Stationary Weight-Bearing Exercises

These exercises encourage the dog to bear weight while standing in place. This is helpful in the early stages of recovery from surgery, when your dog may not want to begin using a previously injured leg.

### ■ *One Leg Standing*

Work with your veterinarian or therapist before performing this exercise. This exercise may be used for problems of either the front or hind legs. Lift the dog's **unaffected** leg. This forces your dog to use the affected leg. Hold for 10 to 15 seconds. Repeat two or three times. Increase the time and repetitions as the dog's strength increases. As the dog gets stronger, she will be able to support herself, with less weight supported by you.

# Active Stretches

### ● *Cervical Flexion*

This exercise is used to encourage your dog to place more weight on the front legs. With the dog standing, hold a treat above your dog's head; then hold a treat between his front legs, at the chest. Resist giving the treat for 5 to 10 seconds, to get your dog to hold the stretch.

### ● *Spine Flexion*

This exercise is used to encourage your dog to place more weight on the hind legs. With your dog standing, hold a treat at your dog's front toes. Resist giving the treat for 5 to 10 seconds, to get your dog to hold the stretch.

### ● *Cervical and Thoracic Bend*

This exercise will encourage your dog to bear weight on the side opposite the side where you hold the treat. With your dog standing, hold a treat behind the shoulder blade. Resist giving the treat for 5 to 10 seconds, to get your dog to hold the stretch.

### ● *Full Bend*

This will encourage your dog to bear weight on the side opposite the side you are holding the treat. With your dog

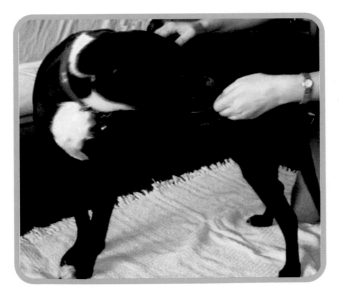

standing, hold a treat at the dog's hip. Resist giving the treat for 5 to 10 seconds, to get your dog to hold the stretch.

### ■ Balance Board

Work with your veterinarian or therapist before performing this exercise.

Balance board exercise can help your dog regain stability and reflexes. Benefits include:

- **Improved balance and coordination**
- **Better reflexes for injury prevention**
- **Greater trunk and pelvic girdle stability**
- **Increased leg and ankle motion**

The balance board is usually 20 inches square, with a 14-degree angle of tilt. Homemade versions may vary from these specifications, but they're still suitable.

**Using the Board** Position your dog's front feet centrally over the board, shoulder width apart. Begin by slowly moving the board, front to back, for 20 repetitions. Support your dog as needed. Be sure to keep the rocking motion under control. Next, lift your dog, rotate the board 90 degrees, and rock from side to side for 20 repetitions. Your dog will contract and relax his muscles and shift his weight to stay on the board. If your dog is small, you can place the entire dog on the board.

# Moving Exercises

These exercises encourage your dog to bear weight during movement and to begin increasing the demand on the muscles and joints that are required during normal activity.

### ● Slow Walking

One of the best early exercises is slow walking, but it must be done properly to help your dog. Don't make the common mistakes of keeping the lead too tight or, worse yet, allowing the dog to pull, both of which keep your dog from moving normally. The goal is to have your dog bear 100% of his own weight. Another common mistake is walking the dog too fast. If your dog begins to hop or limp noticeably, slow your pace until your dog is walking more normally.

You can increase the time spent walking as your dog gets stronger. Walking on different surfaces (carpet, pavement, short grass, packed sand) can benefit your dog's reflexes.

Try adding circles to the walk. Always keep your dog on the outside (dog on your left for circles to the right, dog on your right for circles to the left) to prevent abnormal movement of your dog's hind end.

### ● *Serpentine*

Walk your dog in a serpentine fashion—on an S-shaped path. Begin with big curves and make the curves tighter as your dog gets stronger and more flexible. Be sure to work your dog more in the direction of its weaker side.

### ■ *Cavalletti Exercises*

Cavalletti poles can be used to increase range of motion, stride length, and stance time.

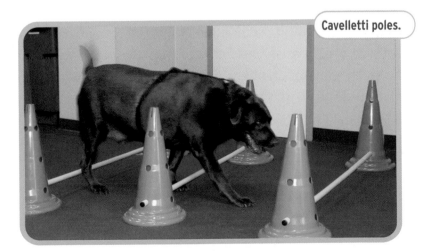

Cavelletti poles.

Start with poles approximately the same distance apart as the height of your dog's elbow. Walk your dog over the poles. You can raise or lower the poles or spread them apart to get the gait you want.

# Rear-Leg Exercises

### ● *Sit to Stand*

Place your dog in a sitting position, by command or with assistance. Hold a treat at the level that your dog's head will be when the dog stands. Ask the dog to stand.

### ● *Down to Stand*

Place the dog in a "sphinx down" position by command or with help. Hold a treat where your dog's head will be when the dog stands. Ask the dog to stand.

### ● *Incline*

Walk your dog up hills or inclines, gradually increasing the grade.

# Front-Leg Exercises

### ■ *Wheelbarrow*

Lift both of your dog's rear legs and hold them for 10 to 15 seconds. Repeat two to three times. Increase the time and number of repetitions as the dog's strength increases. Don't lift the dog too high off the ground, because this can cause discomfort. When your dog is strong enough that he no longer has trouble supporting himself in the stationary position, begin walking slowly forward while holding both of the dog's rear legs. Begin with two or three steps and increase until your dog can move forward 10 steps.

### ● *Down to Sit*

Start with the dog in the "down" position. Lure the dog to a sitting position by raising your hand above the dog's head.

## ■ *Physioroll or Physioball*

Hold the leg opposite the injured leg and roll the dog forward. The dog will reach for the ground with the injured leg. Gently bounce the dog while the leg is on the ground.

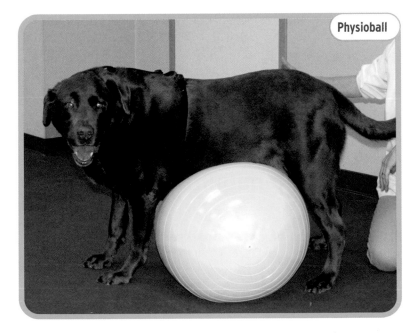

Physioball

## ● *Trail of Treats*

Place treats on the floor about a foot apart. Allow your dog to walk slowly, sniffing the ground. This keeps the dog's weight over the feet and encourages the dog to bear weight on both front feet.

## ■ *Decline*

Walk the dog down hills or a ramp to encourage her to bear weight on the front legs.

## ■ *Tunnel*

Walking through a tunnel, the dog will crouch, causing increased weight bearing on the front legs.

# Rehabilitation Methods and Exercises for Osteoarthritis

The following section lists the methods and exercises that can be used for specific joints. You can perform some of the exercises—these preceded by a green circle—at home with verbal instruction only. Others—those preceded by a yellow square—you should perform at home only after being trained by a rehabilitation therapist. Finally, some—those preceded by a red triangle—must be performed only by a trained rehabilitation therapist in a clinic environment.

## Rear-Leg Rehabilitation Program
*Hip*

**PROBLEM:** *Loss of extension (range of motion)*

**EXERCISES**
- Passive range of motion
- Active range of motion
- Cavalletti
- Walking in 6 inches of high grass
- Walking in 6 inches of water

**PROBLEM:** *Loss of pelvic muscle mass*

**EXERCISES**
*Stationary weight-bearing exercises*
- One leg standing
- Cross-leg standing
- Sit to stand
- Down to stand

*Moving weight-bearing exercises*
- Slow walking
- Incline
- ▲ Underwater treadmill
- Serpentine walking

**PROBLEM:** *Muscle guarding (your dog shies away from your touch because of pain)*

**EXERCISES**
- Physioball
- Active stretching
- Balance board

**METHODS**
- Massage therapy
- ▲ Therapeutic ultrasound
- ▲ Electrical stimulation for pain control

## Knee or Stifle

**PROBLEM:** *Loss of range of motion*

**EXERCISES**
- Passive range of motion
- Active range of motion
- Cavalletti
- ● Walking in 6 inches of high grass
- ● Walking in 6 inches of water

**PROBLEM:** *Loss of foreleg muscle*

**EXERCISES**

*Stationary weight-bearing exercises*
- One leg standing
- Cross-leg standing
- Down to sit

*Moving weight-bearing exercises*
- Slow walking
- Decline
- ▲ Underwater treadmill
- ● "Trail of Treats"
- Serpentine walking

**PROBLEM:** *Muscle guarding*

**EXERCISES**
- Physioball
- Active stretching
- Balance board

## METHODS

- ■ Massage therapy
- ▲ Therapeutic ultrasound
- ▲ Electrical stimulation for pain control

### Ankle or Hock

**PROBLEM:** *Loss of extension (range of motion)*

## EXERCISES

- ■ Passive range of motion
- ■ Active range of motion
- ■ Cavalletti
- ● Walking in 6 inches of high grass
- ● Walking in 6 inches of water
- ▲ Underwater treadmill

**PROBLEM:** *Muscle guarding*

## EXERCISES

- ■ Physioball
- ■ Active stretching
- ■ Balance board

## METHODS

- ■ Massage therapy
- ● Therapeutic ultrasound
- ● Electrical stimulation for pain control

# Front-Leg Rehabilitation Program
## Shoulder

**PROBLEM:** *Loss of extension (range of motion)*

## EXERCISES

- ■ Passive range of motion
- ■ Active range of motion
- ■ Cavalletti
- ● Walking in 6 inches of high grass
- ● Walking in 6 inches of water

**PROBLEM: *Loss of shoulder cuff muscle***

**EXERCISES**
*Stationary weight-bearing exercises*
▨ One leg standing
▨ Cross-leg standing
▨ Down to sit

*Moving weight-bearing exercises*
▨ Slow walking
▨ Decline
▲ Underwater treadmill
▨ Tunnel
● "Trail of Treats"

**PROBLEM: *Muscle guarding***

**EXERCISES**
▨ Physioball
▨ Active stretching
▨ Balance board

**METHODS**
▨ Massage therapy
▲ Therapeutic ultrasound
▲ Electrical stimulation for pain control

*Elbow*

**PROBLEM: *Loss of range of motion***

**EXERCISES**
▨ Passive range of motion
▨ Active range of motion
▨ Cavalletti
● Walking in 6 inches of high grass
● Walking in 6 inches of water

**PROBLEM: *Loss of arm muscle***

**EXERCISES**
*Stationary weight-bearing exercises*
▨ One leg standing
▨ Cross-leg standing

- Down to sit
- Wheelbarrow
- Physioball

**Moving weight-bearing exercises**
- Slow walking
- Decline
▲ Underwater treadmill
- Wheelbarrow

## PROBLEM: *Muscle guarding*

### EXERCISES
- Physioball
- Active stretching
- Balance board

### METHODS
- Massage therapy
▲ Therapeutic ultrasound
▲ Electrical stimulation for pain control

## *Wrist (Carpus)*

### PROBLEM: *Loss of range of motion*

### EXERCISES
- Passive range of motion
- Active range of motion
- Cavalletti
● Walking in 6 inches of high grass
● Walking in 6 inches of water
▲ Underwater treadmill

### PROBLEM: *Hyperextension*

### EXERCISES
▲ Underwater treadmill

## Obesity

**PROBLEM:** *Exercise intolerance*

### EXERCISES
▲ Underwater treadmill
◼ Slow walking

**PROBLEM:** *Joint pain*

### EXERCISES
◼ Physioball
◼ Active stretching
◼ Balance board
◼ Underwater treadmill

### METHODS
◼ Massage therapy
▲ Electricalstimulation for pain control
▲ Therapeutic ultrasound

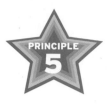
PRINCIPLE
5

# Medications for Osteoarthritis

The fifth principle of the medical management of osteoarthritis is the use of medications. Anti-inflammatory medications are often used to treat osteoarthritis in dogs. You may hear these drugs referred to as NSAIDs, which stands for "nonsteroidal anti-inflammatory drugs." In most cases these medications can do wonders to improve your dog's quality of life and his or her ability to get around, but NSAIDs are not the best treatment for every dog, and some dogs that receive NSAIDs will have mild or, rarely, severe side effects. In this chapter we cover the basics of the use of NSAIDs for osteoarthritis in dogs, including their safety. We also discuss other medications for osteoarthritis such as steroids, opiates, and injectable drugs such as polysulfated glycosaminoglycans (PSGAGs) and hyaluronan.

## What Are Anti-inflammatory Medications?

Nonsteroidal anti-inflammatory drugs, or **NSAIDs,** are the most-prescribed medications for osteoarthritis in dogs, just as they are in people. This class of drugs is known for reducing pain, inflammation, and fever in a variety of conditions. NSAIDs slow the production of chemicals called **prostaglandins,** which cause pain and damage the joints. Prostaglandins cause the pain of osteoarthritis

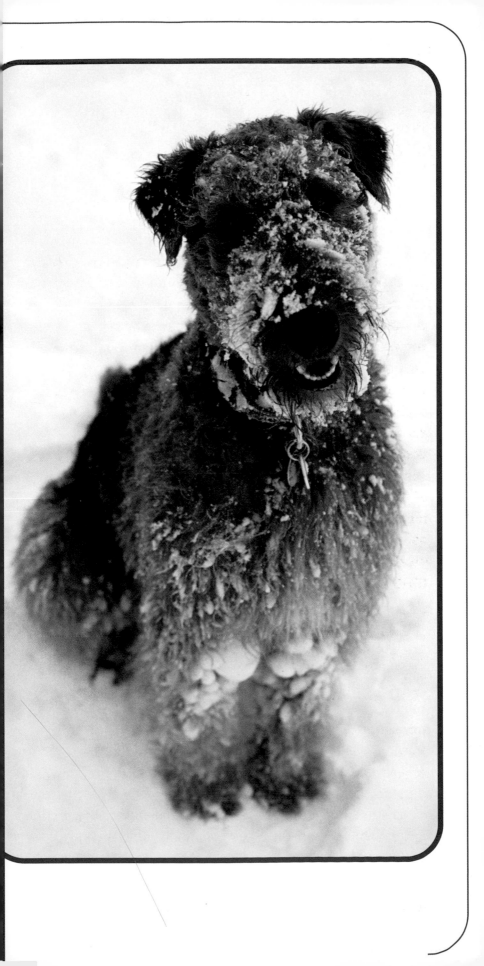

## All About Aspirin

Aspirin, the best-known anti-inflammatory drug, works by blocking cyclooxygenase (COX). There are two types of cyclooxygenase: COX-1, which is always present, and COX-2, which is produced in situations such as disease or trauma.

COX-1 produces prostaglandins that help protect the stomach, kidneys, and blood vessels. COX-2 is thought to be involved more in the production of the prostaglandins associated with pain and inflammation. This explains why taking aspirin gives us pain relief but may also cause an upset stomach.

The ideal anti-inflammatory drug would allow the body to make protective prostaglandins but block the formation of inflammatory prostaglandins. These drugs are referred to as COX-2-specific or COX-2-selective. Debate continues regarding the COX-2 selectivity of individual drugs, but progress has been made in designing drugs that are effective against pain but still safe.

by irritating the surfaces of joints, which causes joints to deteriorate and stimulates the nerve endings.

The best-known NSAID is aspirin (acetylsalicylic acid), a drug most of us are familiar with, but the number of NSAIDs designed and marketed for dogs has increased quite a lot in recent years. This increased availability and marketing of NSAIDs, combined with the fact that NSAIDs for dogs can't always be given to people and vice versa, mean that it is important for you as a dog owner to understand how to use these medications.

Aspirin and phenylbutazone (Butazolidin) were the first anti-inflammatory drugs used commonly in dogs. They're not prescribed as much now because better, safer drugs are available, but they're still useful in certain situations. The newer drugs appear to be safer for most patients, but dog owners should remember that an adverse reaction to any drug can occur in any dog. So you should be alert for any change in your dog's appetite or behavior that could signal an adverse event.

## How Do Anti-Inflammatory Medications Work?

**Arachidonic acid**, a fatty acid found in cell walls, is essential in a dog's diet. When inflammation begins, arachidonic acid is broken down by **cyclooxygenase** into **prostaglandins** and by **lipoxygenase** into **leukotrienes**. This breakdown is known as the inflammatory cascade. Prostaglandins promote swelling and increase the sensitivity of nerves to pain. Leukotrienes attract inflammatory cells that make the inflammation worse and also add to nerve sensitivity. Anti-inflammatory medications block the cyclooxygenase and/or the lipoxygenase from forming prostaglandins and/or leukotrienes, which in turn decreases the pain, swelling, and other characteristics of inflammation. We know there are at least two forms of the cyclooxygenase enzyme, usually called COX-1 and COX-2. COX-1 is normally present in many tissues, whereas inflammation causes COX-2 levels to increase. At one time it was thought that COX-1 was the "good" enzyme and COX-2 was the "bad" enzyme linked to the pain of inflammation. However, it is now clear that the situation is not so simple as this, and that COX-1 can be associated with pain and that COX-2 has some good activities including crucial roles in normal kidney function and also in repair of injured tissue as part of the healing of inflammation.

## Do NSAIDs Have Risks and Side Effects?

Keep in mind that all of the veterinary NSAIDs can cause side effects in dogs and cats. The most common one is gastrointestinal upset. Obvious signs include loss

## What's in a Name?

Drug companies that manufacture anti-inflammatory medications are trying to find drugs that target cycloogygenase-2 (COX-2) and spare cyclooxygenase-1 (COX-1). The description of these drugs has led to some confusion, but the main concern is how much a drug is **stomach protective.** We prefer the term "COX-1 sparing," which suggests that the drug targets COX-2 and lessens the effect on COX-1 and, in this way, lessens harmful effects on the stomach.

Carprofen, meloxicam, deracoxib, and etodolac are all considered COX-1-sparing drugs.

Commonly used terms for COX-2 drugs are:

COX-2 specific

COX-1 sparing

COX-2 preferential

of appetite (anorexia); vomiting; diarrhea; dark, tarry, or bloody stools; and constipation. Kidney or liver disease may appear in some dogs given NSAIDs. A dog with kidney-related side effects may drink more water and urinate more than usual. Signs of side effects involving the liver include yellowing of the gums, skin, or eyes (also known as jaundice). Other side effects include loss of coordination, seizures, sleepiness and lack of energy, shedding, hot spots, and behavior changes. Side effects are rare, though, and most are minor. Most dogs will recover quickly if the medication is stopped for a few days. But if your dog is taking an NSAID and starts to have side effects, be sure to report them to your veterinarian, who will tell you how to care for your pet.

Some NSAIDs also reduce the activity of platelets, which are responsible in part for blood clotting. Aspirin in particular is known to do this, and treatment with aspirin has a dramatic effect on bleeding. It's always a good idea to have routine blood work performed on your dog before your veterinarian prescribes an NSAID, mostly to rule out any existing problems with the kidneys or liver. Dogs with kidney, liver, or stomach disease should never be given NSAIDs without strict veterinary supervision.

Some of the newer human NSAIDs have been linked to heart attacks and other heart problems, and at least one of these drugs was withdrawn from sale. These complications may be less of a concern in dogs, since dogs seem to have far fewer problems than people with the underlying cause of heart attacks: a problem with blood flow to the heart. But, as with all medications, you and your vet-

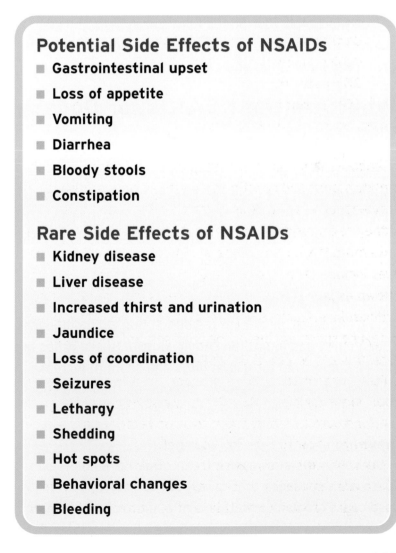

## Potential Side Effects of NSAIDs
- **Gastrointestinal upset**
- **Loss of appetite**
- **Vomiting**
- **Diarrhea**
- **Bloody stools**
- **Constipation**

## Rare Side Effects of NSAIDs
- **Kidney disease**
- **Liver disease**
- **Increased thirst and urination**
- **Jaundice**
- **Loss of coordination**
- **Seizures**
- **Lethargy**
- **Shedding**
- **Hot spots**
- **Behavioral changes**
- **Bleeding**

erinarian should work together closely to be sure that there is no reason your dog should not take a new medication and to be sure that the new drug won't interact with anything else the dog is taking.

Don't forget: If your dog is taking an NSAID and you suspect that your dog is experiencing a side effect, stop giving the medication and call your veterinarian.

# What Are the NSAIDs for Dogs?
## Older NSAIDs

Aspirin and phenylbutazone (Butazolidin) were the first commonly used anti-inflammatory drugs in dogs. These medications are not used as often now because better, safer drugs are available. Because older NSAIDs can cause stomach ulcers, they should be used cautiously in dogs with pain and orthopedic problems.

Although many references supply suggested dog dosages for naproxen (Aleve, Naprosen), meclofenamic acid (Fenamate), piroxicam (Feldene), flunixin meglumine (Banamine), and ibuprofen (Advil, Motrin), these drugs are not FDA approved for use in dogs and seem to increase the likelihood of ulcers, so we discourage their use and will not be discussing them again in this book.

### Aspirin

Although we know aspirin is an effective pain reliever in dogs, the dosages that give relief to your dog often also cause stomach upset, loss of appetite, and vomiting.

Different types of aspirin products are available, including time-release and coated versions, but they haven't gotten rid of the problem of stomach upset.

### How It Works

Aspirin inhibits two types of cyclooxygenase (COX-1 and COX-2), decreasing the production of prostaglandins. In this way it reduces the prostaglandins that cause inflammation and pain (COX-2), but it also stops production of prostaglandins that protect the stomach and kidneys (COX-1). Aspirin also reduces the amount of another prostaglandin (thromboxane) that is involved with platelet function and the formation of blood clots. This is why aspirin is given to people with clotting problems or heart disease. Reduced blood clotting can be helpful to a dog with osteoarthritis, because small clots may actually form in the scar tissue around arthritic joints, but too much aspirin can cause bleeding problems in other places in the body. This is why aspirin is usually stopped about 2 weeks before surgery.

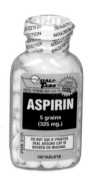

### Dosage

In dogs, aspirin is usually prescribed at a dose of 15 to 25 mg/kg (7 to 12 mg/lb) body weight every 12 hours. The higher dosage should be given for only one or two doses. The dosage should then be reduced to the lowest possible level at which the dog still benefits from the drug. Aspirin should be given with food; although aspirin preparations with stomach protectants may be helpful, often they don't prevent stomach upset.

### Side Effects

The main side effects of aspirin are stomach upset and ulcers. Your veterinarian may give your dog other medications to treat or help prevent ulcers (omeprazole [Prilosec], misoprostol [Cytotec], sucralfate [Carafate]), but it's usually better to switch to another anti-inflam-

## Aspirin

**Mechanism** COX-1 and COX-2 inhibitor
**Dosage** 15 to 25 mg/kg (7 to 12 mg/lb) body weight every 12 hours (limit usage of the higher dose)
**Side effects**

### Common
- Stomach upset

### Rare
- Bleeding
- Liver disease
- Kidney disease

matory medication. Since it cuts down on clotting, aspirin can increase your dog's tendency to bleed, so it should not be given with other medications that prolong bleeding time (polysulfated glycosaminoglycans, for example). A dog receiving one NSAID should never be given another type of NSAID during the same period, because the double dosage puts the dog at a high risk of gastrointestinal problems and other complications. To lower the risk of side effects when switching your dog from aspirin to another pain reliever, wait 2 weeks between the last dose of aspirin and the first dose of the new medication.

### New Veterinary NSAIDs
#### Carprofen
Carprofen was the first new-generation NSAID marketed for dogs in the United States. Marketed under the

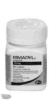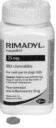

trade name Rimadyl, it's manufactured by Pfizer. Carprofen has been given to more than 10 million dogs in the United States.

### How It Works

Carprofen inhibits COX-2 more than it does COX-1, so it's considered a COX-1–sparing drug. Carprofen's peak effect occurs 1 to 3 hours after the drug is given orally.

### Dosage

Carprofen is useful in treating the pain and inflammation of osteoarthritis in dogs. It also relieves pain associated with surgery and other conditions. The drug is available as caplets, chewable tablets, or an injectable solution. Carprofen may be given orally at a dosage of 2.2 mg/kg (1 mg/lb) twice a day or 4.4 mg/kg (2 mg/lb) once a day. The injectable form is for veterinary use during surgery.

### Side Effects

Side effects of carprofen, which usually involve gastrointestinal upset or ulcers, are rare. A dog given carprofen has a less than 1-in-1000 chance of stomach upset. Most of the time stomach upset is mild, but in rare cases it may be the result of liver damage (hepatopathy). The risk of hepatopathy caused by carprofen is approximately 1 in 5000. At first it was believed that hepatopathy was more common in Labrador retrievers, but this doesn't really seem to be the

## Warning!

NEVER give aspirin or other nonprescription pain relievers while you're giving your dog other NSAIDs. The combination makes it likely that your dog will have gastrointestinal or other complications.

case. Hepatopathy can be fatal, and the first signs are difficult to tell from simple stomach upset. Hepatopathy usually happens during the first 3 weeks a dog is receiving carprofen, but the possibility never goes away completely as long as the dog is receiving the drug. We recommend, as we do with all NSAIDs, that blood work be repeated 1 to 3 months after the medication is started and then again every 6 months to a year. Even though they are rare, side effects on the kidneys have also been reported.

### Deracoxib

Deracoxib, another effective NSAID, is marketed under the trade name Deramaxx by Novartis Animal Health.

#### How It Works

Deracoxib inhibits COX-2 more than it does COX-1, so it's considered a COX-1-sparing drug.

#### Dosage

Deracoxib is available as a chewable tablet. The drug is used to treat acute pain, such as the kind a dog experiences after surgery, at a dose of 3 to 4 mg/kg (1.3 to 2 mg/lb) once a day for up to 7 days.

## Deracoxib

**Mechanism** COX-1-sparing
**Dosage** 1 to 2 mg/kg (0.5 to 1 mg/lb) once a day
**Side effects**

### Rare
- **Stomach upset**

### Very Rare
- **Liver disease**
- **Kidney disease**

When deracoxib is prescribed for chronic pain, such as arthritis pain, the dose is 1 to 2 mg/kg (0.5 to 1 mg/lb) once a day.

### Side Effects

Side effects with deracoxib are rare, with vomiting, diarrhea, and loss of appetite as the most common problems. As with any NSAID, deracoxib should not be given to dogs with known diseases of the stomach, kidney, or liver. The COX-2 enzyme plays a normal role in the function of the kidneys, but this protection is limited with drugs that block COX-2. For dogs without kidney disease, this is rarely a problem; however, as with all NSAIDs, deracoxib should not be given to dogs with kidney disease or those that are dehydrated.

### Etodolac

Etodolac, a Fort Dodge product marketed under the name Etogesic, has been found useful in relieving the clinical signs of osteoarthritis.

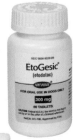

# Etodolac

**Mechanism** COX-1-sparing
**Dosage** 10 to 15 mg/kg (5 to 7 mg/lb) every 24
  hours
**Side effects**

## Rare
- Stomach upset

## Very Rare
- Liver disease
- Kidney disease
- Dry eye

### How It Works
Because etodolac blocks production of COX-2 more than it does COX-1, it's considered a COX-1-sparing drug. It may have other anti-inflammatory effects as well.

### Dosage
Etodolac, which is available as a nonchewable tablet, is administered at a dosage of 10 to 15 mg/kg (5 to 7 mg/lb) every 24 hours.

### Side Effects
Side effects with etodolac are rare and are typical of those seen with the NSAID class of drugs, with vomiting, diarrhea, and loss of appetite being the most common problems. Etodolac may also cause "dry eye" (keratoconjunctivitis sicca), which can seriously affect the eyes if this condition is not recognized and treated early.

## Meloxicam

Meloxicam, a more recently released NSAID, is marketed as Metacam by Boehringer-Ingelheim (it's distributed by Merial in the United States). It's approved for the treatment of postoperative pain in dogs.

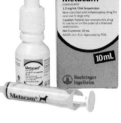

### How It Works

Meloxicam prevents the formation of COX-2 more than it does COX-1, so it is considered a COX-1-sparing drug.

### Dosage

Oral and injectable forms of meloxicam are available. The oral form can be put on your dog's food or placed directly into the dog's mouth. The dose for dogs is 0.1 mg/kg (0.05 mg/lb) once a day. A loading dose of 0.2 mg/kg (0.1 mg/lb) can be given on the first day. It is very

## Where We Stand

We don't really recommend one NSAID over another. Not every NSAID is right for every dog. Some dogs have good results with one NSAID but not another. Some dogs will have side effects with one drug but not another. Some dogs won't benefit from any NSAID and others will have side effects with any of these drugs, but most dogs will benefit from NSAIDS with no side effects. It's important for you to work with your veterinarian to try several of the medications to find the one that works best.

## Meloxicam

**Mechanism** COX-1-sparing
**Dosage** 0.1 mg/kg (0.05 mg/lb) once a day
**Side effects**

### Rare
- **Stomach upset**

### Very Rare
- **Liver disease**
- **Kidney disease**

easy to calculate the correct dose of oral meloxicam: 1 drop per pound of body weight. This is especially useful in small dogs. The injectable form (5 mg/mL) is administered at a dosage of 0.2 mg/kg (0.1 mg/lb), intravenously or subcutaneously. This is equivalent to giving 1 mL for every 55 lb of body weight for the first dose. If another dose is given, it should be only half of the first dose. The oral form may be used after 24 hours at a dosage of 0.1 mg/kg (0.05 mg/lb) once a day.

### Side Effects

Side effects with meloxicam are rare and are typical of those seen with the NSAID class of drugs, with vomiting, diarrhea, and loss of appetite being the most common problems. Meloxicam appears to stay in the body longer than most NSAIDs. If you must switch your dog to another medication, wait about a week after the last dose of meloxicam.

## Tepoxalin

**Mechanism** dual pathway inhibitor
**Dosage** 10 mg/kg (5 mg/lb) once a day
**Side effects**

### Rare
- Stomach upset

### Very Rare
- Liver disease
- Kidney disease

### Tepoxalin

Tepoxalin was recently released by Schering-Plough as a treatment for pain and inflammation associated with osteoarthritis. It is marketed under the name Zubrin.

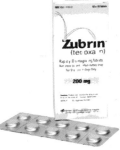

#### How It Works

Tepoxalin inhibits two types of enzymes that can promote osteoarthritis: cyclooxygenase and lipoxygenase, which leads to the production of both prostaglandins and leukotrienes. Inhibiting both pathways can help reduce the pain of osteoarthritis and may also help reduce the risk of gastrointestinal ulceration that can be associated with inhibition of cyclooxygenase. It remains to be seen whether it provides an advantage over the cyclooxygenase inhibitors in dogs with osteoarthritis.

#### Dosage

The drug comes as a rapidly disintegrating tablet that dissolves in the mouth within 4 seconds, although owners often choose to give the tablet in food. The label dose is

10 mg/kg (5mg/lb) orally once a day. Occasionally a veterinarian may recommend a higher dose of 20 mg/kg (10 mg/lb) on the first day of treatment only, if the veterinarian judges the patient to be suffering more severe pain.

### Side Effects

Side effects with tepoxalin are rare and are typical of those seen with the NSAID class of drugs, with vomiting, diarrhea, and loss of appetite being the most common problems.

## Can I Give My Dog NSAIDs If She Is Getting Other Drugs?

Although NSAIDs are safe in combination with many other drugs, certain medications, including steroids and other NSAIDs, should never be given at the same time as NSAIDs. The combination of these medications can have severe and often fatal effects on the stomach, liver, or kidneys. Wait at least 48 hours between the last dose of the old NSAID and the first dose of a new one. A longer wait-

## Where We Stand

NSAIDs should be used when they significantly improve quality of life. Because of the potential side effects and long-term effects of NSAIDs, they are always used at the lowest dose possible and only as needed. But most dogs will have no side effects or long-term effects from these drugs. Proper use of NSAIDs includes observation for positive effects of the medication, along with regular monitoring of blood work (every 6 to 9 months) to check for potential harmful effects.

ing time may be needed if the dog has had any evidence of side effects with the previously administered NSAID.

When giving your dog aspirin, don't give any other medications that will prolong bleeding time.

Some NSAIDs have unique interactions with other medications, such as antibiotics. Always check with your veterinarian if your dog is going to be getting more than one prescription medication at a time.

## Can I Give My Dog NSAIDs Designed for Human Use?

Many of the NSAIDs people take are poisonous, even fatal, in dogs. Such drugs have no real advantages over the veterinary NSAIDs, and their safety in dogs is not known—so they should never be given to dogs.

## How Do I Tell Whether My Dog Needs an NSAID?

NSAIDs are often prescribed for pain control after surgery or for chronic pain in joint disease. Because of their side effects, NSAIDs are always used at the lowest

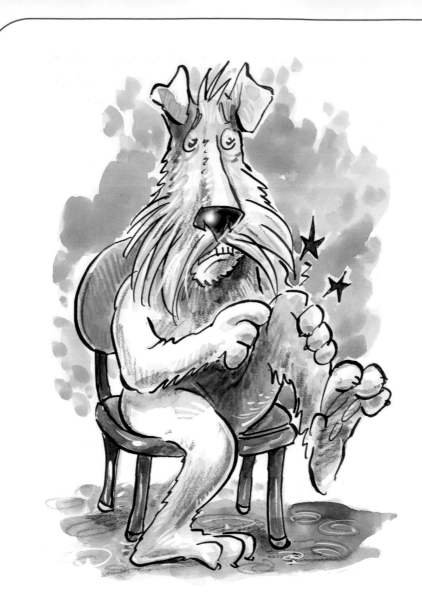

dosage possible, but because side effects are rare, you should feel comfortable giving your dog NSAIDs under your veterinarian's supervision.

The best way to tell whether your dog needs NSAIDs is to conduct a "clinical trial" in your home. Use one of the medications for 2 to 3 weeks and watch your dog for improvement in quality of life and function. Can your dog go on longer walks? Is your dog more interested in playing?

Does the dog find it easier to get up? Keeping a brief diary will help you and your veterinarian decide whether the medication is helping ease your dog's pain (see Appendix G).

## How Should NSAIDs Be Used?

In some cases, certain NSAIDs are used to treat specific forms of cancer, but the most common uses are in the treatment of pain after surgery and in the treatment of chronic osteoarthritis pain.

There are several ways to give your dog an NSAID. The first is to give the NSAID only when your dog seems to be in pain. For this method, you would give your dog a specific dosage once or twice when your dog showed signs of pain. This is a good way to use NSAIDs in a dog that only rarely has pain. It is not very useful in dogs with long-term constant pain, nor is it useful in dogs that tend to hide their discomfort.

Another way to use this method is to also give the medication before you expect your dog to be in pain. If you know that your dog will be in pain after a weekend hike, give an NSAID before the hike. It is well understood that it's easier to prevent pain than to treat it. By having the medication in the bloodstream at the time of an activity, your dog may have much less pain during and after the exercise.

It is easier to prevent pain than to treat it. If you are using NSAIDs in your dog from time to time, always consider giving a dose of the medicine before the dog starts any vigorous activity instead of waiting until after the dog exhibits pain.

> ## Four Methods of Administration of NSAIDs
>
> 1. Infrequent use as needed for the treatment of pain
> 2. Infrequent use as needed for the prevention of pain.
> 3. Short-term steady use to treat a short-term cause of pain.
> 4. Long-term steady use to treat chronic pain.

A third way of using NSAIDs is to treat pain that is expected to go away over time—for example, pain associated with surgery. NSAIDs are often used for surgical pain, which usually disappears during healing. After soft tissue surgery, the pain might be gone after several days; pain from orthopedic surgery might last weeks. In these cases your veterinarian will prescribe NSAIDs to be given every day for a set amount of time. Even though you may not see signs of continuing pain, call your veterinarian before stopping the NSAID. Remember, most dogs don't show pain easily.

The fourth way to use NSAIDs is to treat chronic pain. The most common causes of long-term pain in dogs are osteoarthritis and cancer. In most of these cases the source of pain is with the dog for the rest of its life, although the level of pain may vary from day to day. In these cases we assume that the dog will have constant pain and we will give pain medication every day on a regular basis.

As long as your dog is not showing any side effects, and regular blood work doesn't turn up any signs of trouble, it's safe to use these medications daily for as long as they're needed. Again, because many dogs do not show pain easily and because it is always easier and better to prevent pain than to treat it, don't hesitate to give these

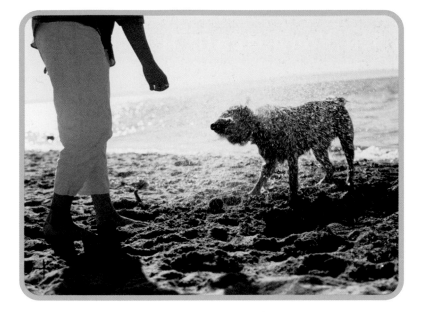

medications as prescribed by your veterinarian. If you think that a medication is no longer necessary or that it's causing side effects, call your veterinarian for advice.

## How Do I Choose an NSAID?

Deciding which NSAID to use gets more complicated as more drugs come on the market. Some of the things to think about include previous success or side effects, your dog's existing medical conditions, which drug your veterinarian prefers to use, and the cost.

If a medication was effective before in easing pain without causing side effects, it's logical to use it again unless something about your dog's health has changed. If a medication was not effective or caused side effects, you

Just because one NSAID doesn't work does not mean that none of them will. In the same way, just because one NSAID causes side effects does not mean that they all will.

# The Home NSAID Trial

1. Identify which NSAIDs may be tried. Recall any earlier use of NSAIDs (whether these drugs were useful or caused complications), and think about your dog's current medical situation.
2. With your veterinarian's help, select an appropriate NSAID and plan to use it for a 2- to 3-week trial period.
3. Keep a record of your dog's activity level, pain versus comfort, and anything you think might be a side effect (stop the medication and call your veterinarian if you think you have seen a side effect). Don't forget to take into account other medications and changes in activity and weight when you assess the effectiveness of a new medication. See Appendix G.
4. If the treatment is working, keep going. Your veterinarian will help you get the dosage as low as possible by doing one of two things (or both, if things are really going well):
   - Decreasing the dosage
   - Decreasing the frequency

If the treatment has not worked, you and your veterinarian will start trying another medication. You should wait at least 48 hours before starting a new medication.

When you find the medication that works and is safe, go back to step 4.

A sample weekly diary is provided in Appendix G to help you track effects and side effects.

> NSAIDs are always given at the lowest dosage and frequency necessary to achieve pain control. You should always consult with your veterinarian before changing the dosage or frequency.

should probably try a different one. It's important to know that just because one NSAID isn't effective doesn't mean that none of them will work, and just because one drug causes side effects in your dog doesn't mean that they all will.

If your dog has a specific medical problem such as liver or kidney disease or bleeding problems, your veterinarian will choose a medication that will not make these problems worse.

The costs of most NSAIDs for dogs are all about the same, except for aspirin, which is quite a bit cheaper. However, as we've discussed, aspirin causes significant side effects in many dogs, and when you add in the costs of other medications used to prevent or treat these side effects, that can make aspirin much more expensive than one of the newer NSAIDs that are made especially for dogs.

In an otherwise healthy dog that has never been given NSAIDs before, the veterinarian will draw on his or her experience and preference to choose a drug. You and your veterinarian have many drugs to choose from, and you almost always will be able to find one that's both effective and safe. We recommend a home trial to help figure out which drug or drugs will work.

Once you and your veterinarian find the right medication, use it at the lowest possible dosage that still controls your dog's pain. Always check with your veterinarian before changing a dosage or frequency, and remember that in most cases you don't have to be concerned about long-term regular use of these medications.

## How Do I Know My Dog Is Not Having Side Effects?

It's important to keep an eye on your dog for side effects of NSAIDs. The first step is to be aware of possible side effects and watch for them. The second step is to record any side effects and call your veterinarian if they occur.

It is also important to monitor your dog for unseen side effects. We recommend complete blood work for most dogs before NSAIDs are started.

If your dog is going to be receiving an NSAID for more than several months, have blood work performed to check liver and kidney function at 3 months and then every 6 months.

## What about Costs?

NSAIDs for dogs are not cheap. The cost of treating a 45-lb (20-kg) dog for 1 month is about $35. Additional costs include visits to the veterinarian and blood work to make sure the drug is not harming your dog.

Ultimately you and your veterinarian must work together to evaluate these costs against the costs of other treatments, such as surgery, that might give your dog relief from pain.

# Other Medications

## Steroids

Steroids are powerful but inexpensive drugs that have been used for many years to treat osteoarthritis in dogs. Unfortunately, these drugs also have powerful and dangerous side effects that can threaten the life of your dog.

Steroids are the drugs of choice in the treatment of **immune-mediated** osteoarthritis in dogs. This type of disease, which has been described in previous chapters, accounts for just a fraction of a percent of all cases of osteoarthritis in dogs. In the immune-mediated form of **arthritis,** the steroids block the process of cartilage destruction. In these cases, steroids are used at high doses for short periods of time (weeks).

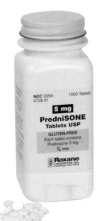

The use of steroids in osteoarthritis is controversial; in fact, most veterinarians and surgeons discourage their use. Steroids often make the arthritic dog feel better for a while. They may also make your dog want to eat, drink, and urinate more. But osteoarthritis is a long-term disease that continues to progress. Long-term use of steroids actually adds to the destruction of cartilage, weakens the muscles and other soft tissues, and disturbs the normal hormone balance. Long-term use of steroids contributes to destruction of the body. The only times steroids are recommended in the treatment of osteoarthritis are when **immune-mediated joint disease** has been identified and when the dog is terminally ill. Otherwise, this quick fix can cause problems much worse than the osteoarthritis itself.

## Where We Stand

Because of the long-term bad effects of steroids on the body and on the joints themselves, we do not support the routine use of steroids in the treatment of osteoarthritis.

# Opiates

Opiates, some of the strongest painkillers known, include such drugs as morphine and butorphanol. Although these drugs are often used to ease pain in hospitalized dogs, usually they can't be sent home with the owner because they are carefully controlled by the government. Some exceptions include oral morphine tablets, fentanyl patches, and butorphanol, which is found in some cough suppressants. Morphine tablets may be sent home only in small amounts because they may be abused by people. Fentanyl patches, which only last about 72 hours, pose a risk in homes with small children. Butorphanol has a very short period of usefulness (45 minutes to an hour), so it would have to be given every hour of the day to control pain. Opiates can have serious side effects, including changes in respiration and heart rate and sedative effects—and dogs can become addicted to opiates just as people do! For these reasons, opiates are not a good choice for long-term pain relief in osteoarthritis and should be used only for short periods under the close supervision of your veterinarian.

## Where We Stand

NSAIDs can be an important and effective part of managing your dog's osteoarthritis pain. But studies support that the best overall treatment is "multimodal," or using multiple methods. Other methods that should always be employed include weight control and exercise moderation. Other methods that may be employed include nutritional supplements, physical rehabilitation, and use of other medications such as tremadol.

### Tremadol

Tremadol is a drug with actions similar to those of opiates, although unlike opiates, it is not controlled by the government. It is used commonly in humans for chronic pain of cancer and is being used more commonly in dogs for pain of cancer and osteoarthritis. Tremadol is usually used at a dosage of 1 to 4 mg/kg (0.5 to 2 mg/lb) two to four times a day. Few side effects have been reported in dogs, although there are no long-term studies to determine if there are risks for prolonged use of this medication. Because of the potential for addiction, the government may increase control of this medication in the future.

### Amantadine

Amantadine acts in the central nervous system to limit pain and has been used for the treatment of severe pain in humans. Amantadine is being investigated as a potential medication for the treatment of osteoarthritis in dogs as part of a "multimodality" approach.

# Other Medical Therapies for Osteoarthritis

Many other medications have been investigated in the treatment of osteoarthritis. Some have been intended for pain control; others are intended to alter the disease itself or aid in the normal function of the joint. We'll discuss two here.

### Polysulfated Glycosaminoglycan (Adequan)

Injectable polysulfated glycosaminoglycan (PSGAG) is marketed as Adequan by Luitpold Pharmaceuticals. PSGAGs are found naturally in joint cartilage. The idea behind the use of PSGAGs is similar to the idea behind the use of **chondroitin sulfate** as a nutritional supplement. In fact, the two molecules are similar except in size. PSGAGs are much larger than chondroitin sulfate. The larger molecule is more like the actual molecules in cartilage, and once it's in the joint, it's more likely to stay there. On the other hand, it's harder to get the larger molecule into the joint to do its work.

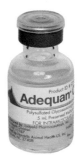

### How It Works

Exactly how Adequan works is not known. In theory, this medication strengthens cartilage to limit further damage and even promotes cartilage healing, but studies have turned up conflicting results, so Adequan alone probably isn't able to cause significant healing.

Adequan does seem to ease pain and improve function in some dogs. It may work in the same way as nutritional supplements such as **glucosamine** and chondroitin. Like these supplements, Adequan may block some of the pathways of inflammation, easing pain and cutting down on inflammation.

Adequan also limits blood clotting. This may be of benefit in osteoarthritis, because small blood clots tend to form in the soft tissues surrounding the joint, leading to greater scar tissue formation. Less clotting could help limit scar tissue and improve the flexibility of arthritic joints. The effects of Adequan on blood clotting probably don't lead to bleeding problems elsewhere in the body, but check with your veterinarian before using any other medication, such as aspirin, that could contribute to increased bleeding.

### Dosage

Adequan has been widely used as an intramuscular injection; studies by its manufacturer suggest that injecting it into muscle results in significant concentrations of the medication in the joint, although this finding is still a matter of controversy. It is usually given in a dosage of 4 mg/kg (2 mg/lb) twice a week for 3 or 4 weeks, not to exceed 8 dosages.

### Side Effects

Adequan doesn't cause any common side effects. In rare cases, a dog may experience stomach upset or other unusual complications. Bleeding is rarely a problem unless Adequan is used in combination with other drugs that contribute to increased bleeding.

### How Do I Know Whether My Dog Needs Adequan?

Whether Adequan is right for your dog depends on many factors, including your veterinarian's experience and preferences, the specific cause of your dog's osteoarthritis, the dog's response to other medications, cost, and convenience.

Adequan is often used when the chance that cartilage will heal is good—for example, when a normal joint is fractured. In osteoarthritis caused by **dysplasia,** the benefit of medications such as Adequan is probably limited to pain control. This is because cartilage healing in these cases is unlikely because of the mechanical factors that are causing the destruction of cartilage.

Adequan may be used as a "first-line drug" or as a supplemental agent for treatment of chronic osteoarthritis and pain. We often use Adequan when nutritional supplementation and NSAIDs are not enough to control pain. In some dogs, Adequan provides improved function and pain relief.

The most significant limitations of Adequan are its cost and convenience. In addition to the cost of the product, your veterinarian may charge for the veterinary visit and the injection. Some clients choose to give the injections themselves, at home.

### How Do I Tell Whether the Adequan Is Working?

The only way to tell for certain that Adequan is working is to watch your dog to see whether his quality of life and function are improving. Using the weekly diary we provide in Appendix G, you can record such functions as stair-climbing, running, and jumping. You can also record your impressions of the degree of pain or discomfort. Remember to consider other factors that may be contributing to improvement, such as changes in medication or weight. We usually recommend a month-long home trial of Adequan.

## Hyaluronan

### What Is Hyaluronan?

Hyaluronan is found naturally in the joint in two locations: as the backbone of a major structure of the cartilage matrix and as one of the most important lubricants in the joint. Just as oil serves as a lubricant in your car's engine, allowing the parts to move smoothly, hyaluronan allows the joint surfaces to move against each other smoothly. In osteoarthritis, the **joint fluid** changes and becomes a

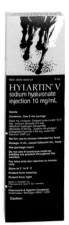

less effective lubricant. The irregular joint surfaces may grind against each other, contributing to the pain of the disease. Hyaluronan can be injected to replace the missing lubrication. Some people report improved function for as long as 6 months. Hyaluronan may have other, still-undetermined effects on the joints.

### Dosage

Hyaluronan is marketed by several companies. Talk to your veterinarian about the specifics of the product that will be used.

Specific dosages have not been determined for dogs. The most common way of using hyaluronan is as an intra-articular injection (given directly into the joint). We recommend one injection every 2 weeks for three injections. The volume injected depends on the size of the joint. The dog must be sedated and the area kept sterile, and the veterinarian must have experience in joint injections.

### Side Effects

Hyaluronan has no common side effects. If the injection is done wrong or the dog has an underlying illness,

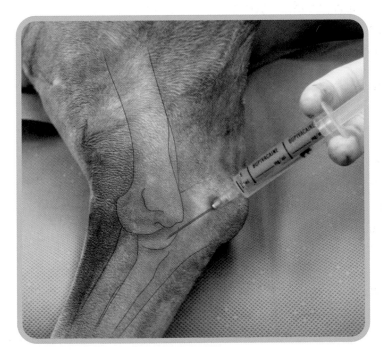

the risk of inflammation or infection associated with the injection may be higher.

### How Do I Know Whether My Dog Needs Hyaluronan?

Whether hyaluronan might work for you and your dog depends on many factors, including the experience and preferences of your veterinarian, the specific cause of your dog's osteoarthritis, the dog's response to other medications, cost, and convenience.

Hyaluronan may be used as an initial treatment or as a supplemental treatment for cases of chronic osteoarthritis and pain. As with Adequan, we often use hyaluronan when nutritional supplements and NSAIDs are not controlling pain well. In some dogs, hyaluronan significantly improves function and relieves pain.

The most significant limitations of hyaluronan are cost and convenience. One treatment may cost as much as $100. You may also be charged for the veterinary visit and the injection.

### How Do I Tell Whether the Hyaluronan Is Working?

The only way to tell for certain whether hyaluronan is working is to watch your dog and observe the dog's quality of life and function. Using the weekly diary we've provided, you can record such functions as stair-climbing, running, and jumping. You can also record your impressions of your dog's degree of pain or discomfort. Remember to consider other factors that may be contributing to improvement, such as changes in medication or weight. We recommend a home trial of hyaluronan for one cycle of three injections. Look for improvement to occur within a few weeks and to last for as long as 6 months. About 50% of dogs will respond positively to hyaluronan.

Now let's review the information in this chapter:

- Nonsteroidal anti-inflammatory drugs, or NSAIDs, are the most widely prescribed medications for osteoarthritis in dogs, just as they are in humans.
- NSAIDs act by reducing the production of chemicals called prostaglandins, which cause pain and damage the joints.
- The most basic NSAID is aspirin.
- NSAIDs that are usually prescribed by veterinarians include Rimadyl (carprofen), Deramaxx (deracoxib), Etodolac (etogesic), Metacam (meloxicam), and Zubrin (tepoxalin).
- NSAIDs have a low likelihood of side effects. The most common ones are vomiting and anorexia ( a loss of appetite or a reluctance to eat) caused by stomach upset; more serious side effects involve the liver and kidneys.
- An NSAID should never be given with another NSAID or with a steroid.
- NSAIDs may be given daily or just whenever they are needed to relieve or prevent pain.
- It is more effective to prevent pain than to treat it.
- Your veterinarian will probably recommend having blood work done every 6 months if your dog is getting NSAIDs on a long-term basis.
- Never give your dog a human medication without first asking your veterinarian.
- Steroids should be used cautiously to treat osteoarthritis.
- Other medications such as hyaluronic acid and Adequan (polysulfated glycosaminoglycan) may help treat osteoarthritis, although this has not been thoroughly proved.

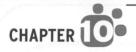

# Basic Surgeries for Osteoarthritis

Veterinary surgery has advanced quite a bit in the past 20 years. Today many surgical options are available for the treatment of osteoarthritis in your dog. These procedures may be performed by your regular veterinarian, but more advanced procedures may require the skills of a surgeon certified through the American College of Veterinary Surgeons.

In this chapter we'll give you a basic introduction to the kinds of surgeries that are available for the treatment of osteoarthritis in dogs. Use this chapter as a reference as you read about the specific treatment of joint diseases in the chapters that follow.

# Issues of Orthopedic Surgery

You, as the owner, are the best person to make decisions about your pet's welfare. Only you understand the role of your dog in your family's life, and only you can make the ethical and financial decisions required when surgery for your pet may be necessary. For this reason, you need to find reliable sources of information. In considering orthopedic surgery for your dog, you should understand:

- **The basic reason for the surgery**
- **The risks of the surgery**
- **The cost of the surgery**
- **The care you will need to provide your dog after the surgery**
- **The expectations for the surgery**

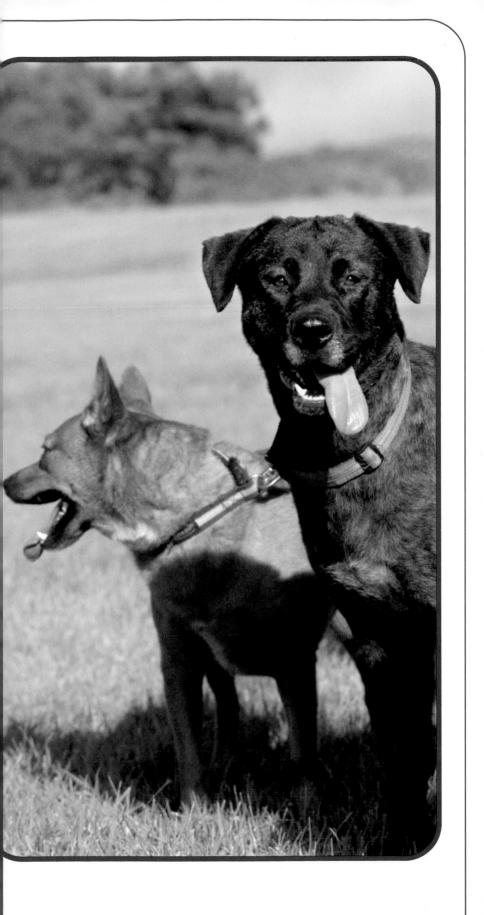

## Where We Stand

We strongly believe that the final decision in the treatment of your pet should be made by you, the owner. The job of the veterinarian and the veterinary surgeon is to provide you with the best information so that you can make the best choice for your particular situation.

This chapter, plus information from your regular veterinarian and your veterinary surgeon, will provide the information you need to make an educated decision that is right for your dog and your family.

# How Do I Know Whether My Dog Needs Surgery for Osteoarthritis?

The decision to go ahead with surgery to treat osteoarthritis is obvious in many cases but may be much more difficult in others. For acute injuries to joints that can be corrected easily, your veterinarian will recommend surgery as the main therapy. In osteoarthritis that results from other causes, especially developmental diseases such as **dysplasia,** the benefits of surgery are still not agreed on, and many factors must be considered. These factors include the severity of the disease, the age of the dog, how well the dog is expected to do after surgery, and the cost of the procedure. The best way to decide on surgery for your dog is to talk to your veterinarian and a board-certified surgeon and to educate yourself using reliable sources of information. Pet owners are most satisfied when they make important health care decisions themselves, rather than asking the veterinarian to decide for them. For this reason, having reliable information is very important.

# Orthopedic Surgery Procedures Used in Osteoarthritis

Many different surgical procedures are performed on dogs to treat osteoarthritis. The most common procedures are listed in the accompanying box.

## Common Surgical Procedures for the Treatment of Osteoarthritis

### Correcting the Cause of Osteoarthritis

Fracture repair—repair of joint fractures is often performed with metal pins, bone screws, and bone plates.

Joint stabilization—unstable joints such as the knee are often repaired by replacing the torn ligament with strong suture or surgical wire.

Correction of "nonmatching" bones (you may hear this described as "incongruity")—joints with incongruity are often treated by an osteotomy. One or more bones are cut and rotated and then repaired with bone plates and screws.

### Alteration of Joint Loading

Tibial plateau leveling osteotomy—in this procedure for ligament rupture in the knee, the tibia or lower bone of the hind limb is cut, rotated, and then repaired with a special bone plate and screws to realign the knee joint.

### Removal of Loose Bodies in Joints

Osteochondritis dissecans (OCD) flap removal—in this disease, a piece of cartilage becomes loose in the joint. The flap must be removed for the joint to heal. The flap may be removed by either arthroscopy or arthrotomy.

## Common Surgical Procedures for the Treatment of Osteoarthritis—cont'd

Elbow dysplasia fragment removal—in this disease, a piece of bone often breaks off in the elbow. The bone fragment must be removed to avoid further damage to the joint.

### Joint Replacement

Hip replacement—the hip is the most common joint replaced in dogs. The ball and socket are replaced with a plastic and metal joint.
Elbow replacement—this is a relatively new and uncommon procedure.

### Joint Excision

Femoral head and neck excision—this is a common treatment for osteoarthritis of the hip of dogs. The ball of the ball and socket joint is cut away.

### Arthrodesis

Arthrodesis, or fusion, of the carpus (wrist) or hock (ankle) joints in dogs can be very successful with only minimal changes in the way the dog moves and complete relief of osteoarthritis pain. Arthrodesis of other joints is less common, with poorer results.

### Amputation

Amputation is a common procedure in dogs for the treatment of cancer but is very rarely used for the treatment of osteoarthritis.

## Less Common Surgical Procedures for the Treatment of Osteoarthritis

### Débridement and Treatment of Damaged Cartilage

In these procedures, the bone and cartilage of the joint are treated to encourage proper healing;

however, normal healing of cartilage is very difficult to achieve.

### Arthroscopic Joint Lavage
In this procedure, the joint is flushed (lavaged) with fluid to decrease the amount of irritating chemicals in the joint. This procedure is commonly performed for joints with infection but is rarely performed and not highly effective for joints with osteoarthritis.

### Joint Resurfacing
These techniques are performed in people and may help heal cartilage.  They are rarely performed in dogs because of the small size of the dog's joints and their limited success. Some of these procedures include:
> Osteochondral grafts
> Tissue culture cell grafts
> Periosteal grafts

Orthopedic surgery procedures can be separated into two broad categories: those in which the joint is repaired and those in which the joint is replaced or removed. Two general methods are used to perform joint surgery. The older, more traditional method is referred to as arthrotomy, and the more modern technique is referred to as arthroscopy. Each has its own benefits and is best in certain situations.

# Arthrotomy
**Arthrotomy** is the surgical opening of a joint. This is the traditional method of performing joint surgery. The soft tissues and the joint are cut open to allow the surgeon access to inside the joint. Once an arthrotomy has been performed, the surgeon can see inside the joint, take biopsy samples, remove diseased tissue, repair or replace **ligaments,** or even replace the joint.

The benefits of arthrotomy include good access to most parts of most joints, the use of traditional surgical equipment, lower cost, and a large "working space" for the surgeon.

The disadvantages include the need for large amounts of tissue to be cut, increased pain, increased risk of infection, and less visibility compared with arthroscopy.

In osteoarthritis, arthrotomy is used:

- **To remove loose cartilage flaps (in osteochondritis dissecans, or OCD)**
- **To remove loose bone chips (in elbow dysplasia—fragmented coronoid process)**
- **To stabilize a joint (in cruciate injury or dislocated kneecap)**
- **To see and treat damaged soft tissues (in meniscal or ligament tears)**
- **Joint replacement**

## Arthroscopy

**Arthroscopy** is a more modern method of exploring a joint that also is used to see the joint during corrective surgery. In this procedure, specialized telescopes and instruments are sent into the joint through small cuts.

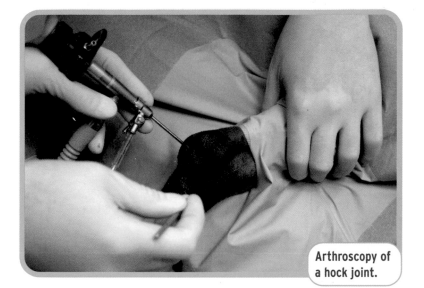

Arthroscopy of a hock joint.

The advantages of arthroscopy are the small cuts that are required to access the joint, less pain, the low risk of infection, and the excellent view (even magnification) of structures inside the joint. Many, but not all, of the procedures that were once performed with arthrotomy can be performed with arthroscopy.

The disadvantages include the need for specialized equipment and training and the increased cost. With some surgical procedures, such as joint replacement, arthrotomy is still required. In the treatment of osteoarthritis, arthroscopy is used:

- **To remove loose cartilage flaps (in OCD)**
- **To remove loose bone chips (in elbow dysplasia–fragmented coronoid process)**
- **To see and treat osteoarthritic areas**
- **To see and treat damaged soft tissues (in meniscal or ligament tears)**

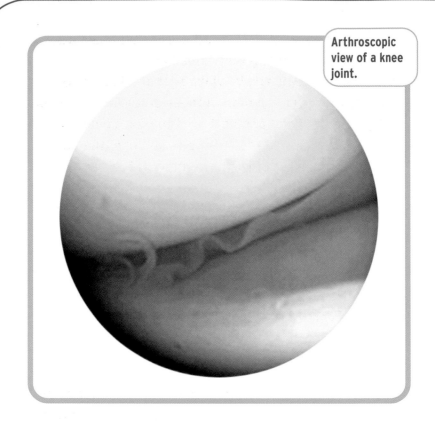

Arthroscopic view of a knee joint.

## Other Common Joint Surgery Procedures

### Arthroplasty

**Arthroplasty** is a general term for any surgical procedure that changes or modifies the structure of a joint. These procedures include:

**Osteotomy.** The term *osteotomy* means to cut bone. In this procedure, the bones are cut and rotated and then repaired using bone plates and screws to realign a joint. Examples of osteotomy include:

Ulnar osteotomy for elbow dysplasia. The ulna or small bone of the forearm is cut and moved to achieve realignment of the elbow joint.

Triple pelvic osteotomy for hip dysplasia. The pelvis is cut in three places, rotated, and then repaired with a special bone plate and screws to realign the hip joint.

Tibial plateau leveling osteotomy for cruciate disease. The tibia or lower bone of the hind limb is cut, rotated, and then repaired with a special bone plate and screws to realign the knee joint.

**Excisional arthroplasty**, in which part of a joint is removed. The most common of these procedures in dogs is the femoral head and neck excision for hip dysplasia. In this procedure, the top of the thigh bone (the ball of the ball and socket of the hip joint) is cut out and discarded.

**Total joint replacement**, in which the joint is removed and replaced with an artificial joint. The most common joint replacement in dogs is the total hip replacement. In this procedure the ball and socket of the hip joint are both replaced with a plastic and metal joint. Total elbow replacements are also becoming more common in dogs.

## Arthrodesis

**Arthrodesis** is the process of permanently immobilizing a joint by converting it to solid bone. It's done only in the most severe cases, when other medical or surgical treatment will not work for any number of reasons. A surgeon performs an arthrodesis by removing the cartilage that remains in the joint and stabilizing the joint with a bone plate or other apparatus until the joint heals to solid bone. The outcome for success with arthrodesis depends mostly on the joint that is being operated on, the size of the dog, and the owner's expectations as to function.

*Shoulder arthrodesis.* This procedure is technically challenging and results in a stiff **gait.**

*Elbow arthrodesis.* This procedure is technically challenging and results in a stiff gait.

*Carpus arthrodesis.* This is a relatively routine procedure; the outcome is usually excellent.

*Hip arthrodesis.* This procedure is not performed; instead, a femoral head and neck excision is performed.

*Knee arthrodesis.* This procedure is technically challenging and results in a stiff gait.

*Hock arthrodesis.* This is a relatively routine procedure; the outcome is usually excellent.

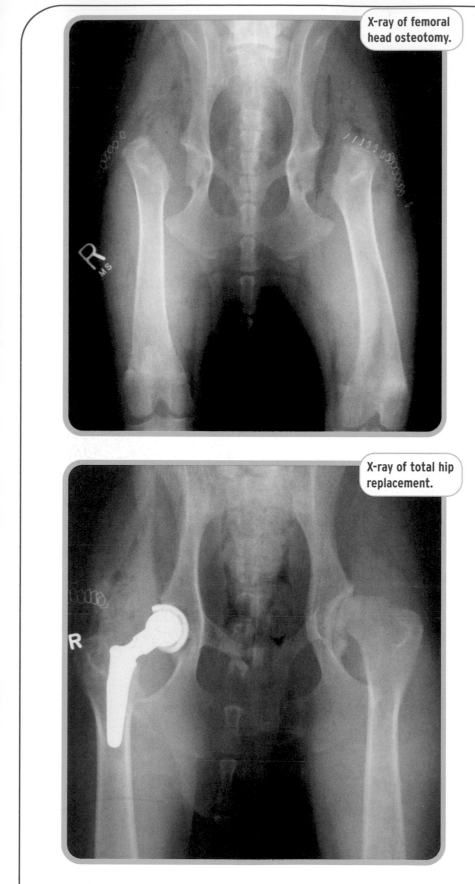

X-ray of femoral head osteotomy.

X-ray of total hip replacement.

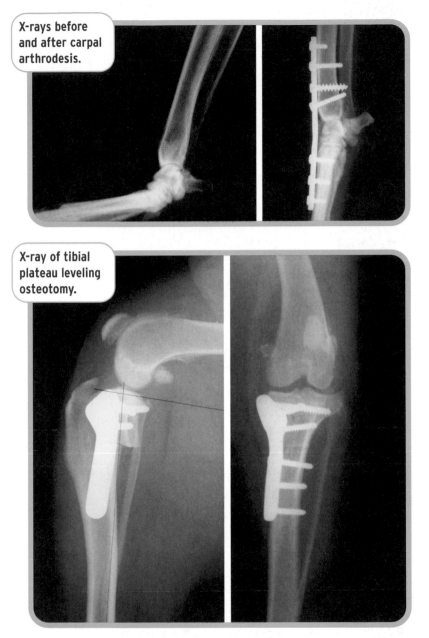

X-rays before and after carpal arthrodesis.

X-ray of tibial plateau leveling osteotomy.

# How Do I Prepare My Dog for Joint Surgery?

Before your dog has surgery, your veterinarian may ask you to stop giving certain medications. If your dog is to have surgery on the day you bring it to the hospital, the hospital staff may ask that you not feed your dog that morning.

Most of your preparation will be for when you bring your dog home. The specific instructions for care after your dog is discharged from the hospital will vary quite a bit, depending on the procedure your dog has and the preferences of your veterinarian. Certain basic principles, however, are always followed when a dog is recovering from bone or joint surgery:

- **Minimizing the risk of injury during the healing period**
- **Watching carefully for complications, including infection, implant failure, and repeat injury**
- **Managing body weight**
- **Administering medications, including analgesics (pain relievers)**
- **Follow-up for reevaluation**

You must follow your veterinarian's discharge instructions for your dog to have a successful outcome. Typical discharge instructions for different orthopedic surgeries are presented in the accompanying boxes.

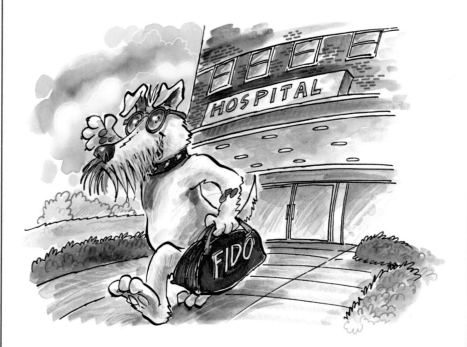

# Example Discharge Instructions for Tibial Plateau Leveling Osteotomy (TPLO)

- Limit movement as directed:
  - Strict exercise restriction until x-rays show adequate healing
  - Leash walking only long enough for urination and defecation
  - No running, jumping, playing, or stair-climbing
- Administer anti-inflammatory analgesics such as Rimadyl (carprofen) or Deramaxx (deracoxib), as directed.
- Apply cold packs to the surgery site for 15 minutes, three times a day, for the first 3 days.
- Call your veterinarian if you see any of the following complications:
  - Swelling of the leg
  - Drainage from the surgery site
  - Opening of the surgery site
  - Poor appetite
  - Signs of severe pain
- Administer nutritional supplements as directed.
- Continue weight-control diet.
- Return for suture removal in 2 weeks.
- Return for x-rays in 6 (range of 6 to 10) weeks.
- Please call your veterinarian if you have any questions.

# Example Discharge Instructions for Arthroscopy

- Limit movement as directed:
  - Strict exercise restriction for the next 4 weeks
  - Leash walking only long enough for urination and defecation
  - No running, jumping, playing, or stair-climbing
- Administer anti-inflammatory analgesics such as Rimadyl (carprofen) or Deramaxx (deracoxib) as directed.
- Apply cold packs to the surgery site for 15 minutes, three times a day, for the first 3 days.
- Call your veterinarian if you see any of the following complications:
  - Swelling of the leg
  - Drainage from the surgery site
  - Opening of the surgery site
  - Poor appetite
  - Signs of severe pain
- Administer nutritional supplements as directed.
- Continue weight-control diet.
- Return for suture removal in 2 weeks.
- Begin home physical therapy as directed or begin physical therapy visits.
- Please call your veterinarian if you have any questions.

# Example Discharge Instructions for Joint Fracture

- Limit movement as directed:
  - Strict exercise restriction until x-rays show adequate healing
  - Leash walking only long enough for urination and defecation
  - No running, jumping, playing, or stair-climbing
- Administer anti-inflammatory analgesics such as Rimadyl (carprofen) or Deramaxx (deracoxib) as directed.
- Apply cold packs to the surgery site for 15 minutes, three times a day, for the first 3 days.
- Call your veterinarian if you see any of the following complications:
  - Swelling of the leg
  - Drainage from the surgery site
  - Opening of the surgery site
  - Poor appetite
  - Signs of severe pain
- Administer nutritional supplements as directed.
- Continue weight-control diet.
- Return for suture removal in 2 weeks.
- Begin home physical therapy as directed or begin physical therapy visits.
- Please call your veterinarian if you have any questions.

## What to Expect after Orthopedic Surgery

Discharge instructions vary from surgeon to surgeon, but the principles are always the same.

- When surgery relies on healing of bone—for example, fracture repair or after an osteotomy (bone cutting)—you must carefully control your dog's activity until the bone is healed. Your veterinarian will almost always verify that your dog's bone is healing using recheck radiographs (x-rays).

- When surgery involves cartilage, you'll need to see that your dog gets both the proper rest and joint motion to be sure that the cartilage is healing but the joint stays mobile. Because cartilage doesn't show up on x-rays, healing cannot be checked on radiographs. Cartilage healing is very limited, but any healing that will occur usually takes place during the first 4 weeks after surgery.

- When surgery involves the healing of a fracture through a joint, rehabilitation must involve both rest (to allow bone and cartilage to heal) and controlled movement (to keep the joint mobile).

Now let's review the information in this chapter:

- In the surgery known as arthrotomy, the joint is cut open.
- In arthroscopy a small viewing scope is sent into the joint through a small cut, and the veterinarian uses the view from this scope to perform surgery.
- In the surgery known as arthrodesis, a joint is permanently fixed in one position.
- In osteotomy, bone is cut, usually to change the forces going through a joint.
- The main risks of orthopedic surgery in dogs are infection, the dangers of anesthesia, and failure of the surgery.
- A successful surgical result depends on restricted exercise and good nursing care during the recuperation period.

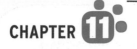

# ALTERNATIVE MEDICINE AND OSTEOARTHRITIS

Alternative and complementary therapies are becoming increasingly popular among people trying to relieve the pain of osteoarthritis. This interest may come from disappointment with poor results of traditional techniques, concern about the side effects of the long-term use of anti-inflammatory medications and about the possible complications of surgery, and increased interest in alternative therapies. The trend is also starting to appear in veterinary medicine, and such treatments as acupuncture and chiropractic are becoming more widely available for pets. However, given the limited information available about the safety and effectiveness of these treatments, it is imperative that dog owners critically evaluate these treatments before using them on their pets.

## Options and Information

Alternative therapies include acupuncture, diets, herbal medicine, **homeopathy,** massage, and **chiropractic** treatment. Although truly scientific information on these therapies is limited, more and more dog owners are considering these therapies in the treatment of their pets' osteoarthritis. A tremendous amount of information is available from such sources as the Internet on alternative therapies and osteoarthritis, but almost none of it represents sound scientific data. Many dog owners pursue these alternative

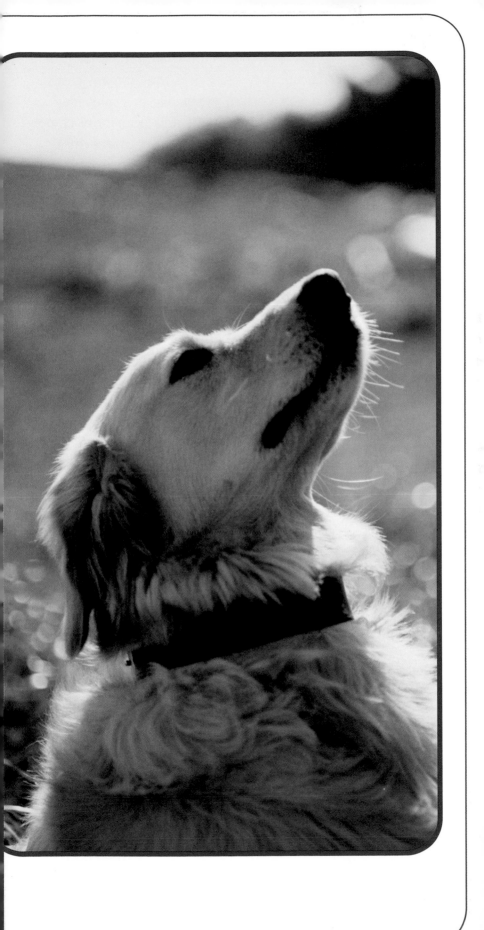

therapies, thinking that they're safer than traditional Western medicine, but they carry risks that in many cases are not explained well. Certain alternative therapies may someday be demonstrated to be effective primary or complementary treatments for the treatment of osteoarthritis, but in the meantime dog owners must ask as many questions as possible of the practitioners of these therapies and talk candidly and openly to their regular veterinarian or surgeon before using them.

# Acupuncture

**Acupuncture** involves the application of small-gauge (thin) needles to specific points on the body in an attempt to treat many different diseases and conditions. It's likely that acupuncture stimulates nerves, alters blood flow, and changes the production of chemical mediators in the body. Acupuncture has been studied most often in the treatment of pain and may be particularly useful in this regard. In people, evidence of the usefulness of acupuncture in the treat-

## Where We Stand

Acupuncture may be an effective way of relieving the pain of osteoarthritis in dogs, but at this time the scientific evidence isn't strong enough for us to recommend acupuncture routinely. We recommend that dog owners considering the use of acupuncture for their pets:

- Always consult with their regular veterinarian or veterinary surgeon first.
- Be certain that the acupuncturist is a licensed veterinarian who is certified in acupuncture.
- Fully understand the risks and expectations of the treatment.

ment of osteoarthritis has been mixed. Acupuncture has been shown to be more effective than placebo treatment in relieving pain, although it has not been shown to be more effective than traditional Western medicine. Acupuncture is probably more effective in treating the pain of osteoarthritis than it is in increasing the flexibility or function of a joint. These results have led to the recommendation that acupuncture be considered a useful complementary therapy in the treatment of osteoarthritis in people.

Acupuncture has been used in China to treat pain and other disorders in animals for more than 4000 years and has been in use in North America for several decades. Only a limited amount of scientific research has been carried out regarding the use of acupuncture for the treatment of osteoarthritis in dogs, but it is probably the most accepted of the alternative therapies. The American Veterinary Medical Association (AVMA) published its position on acupuncture in its *Guidelines for Complementary and Alternative Veterinary Medicine* and states: "Veterinary AP (acupuncture) and acutherapy are considered an integral part of veterinary medicine. These techniques should be regarded as surgical and/or medical procedures under state veterinary practice acts. It is recommended that educational programs be undertaken by veterinarians before they are considered competent to practice veterinary AP."

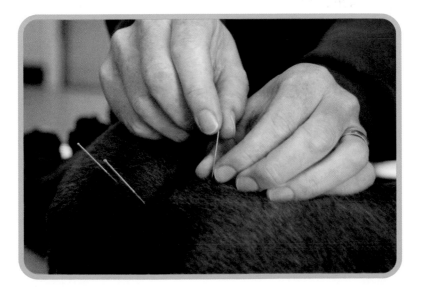

# Where Can I Find Reliable Information on Veterinary Acupuncture?

An excellent resource on the use of acupuncture in animals is available through the American Academy of Veterinary Acupuncture (AAVA) Web site (www.aava.org). The AAVA agrees with the AVMA, stating that a veterinary acupuncturist should be a licensed veterinarian trained and certified in acupuncture. In fact, in most states acupuncture is considered a surgical treatment requiring licensure.

# How Long Do Acupuncture Treatments Take?

Acupuncture appointments generally last 30 minutes to an hour. Some needles are left in place for as little as 10 seconds; others may be kept in the body for as long as 20 minutes.

# How Long Does It Take to See Benefits of Acupuncture?

It is generally accepted that the more chronic the disease, the more treatments are required to see benefits of acupuncture. With an acute joint injury, you may see benefits after one treatment, but because osteoarthritis is a chronic disease, multiple treatments may be necessary before benefits are noticed.

# How Many Treatments Will Be Needed?

It appears that one of the limitations of acupuncture in the management of osteoarthritis is that the benefits are not permanent. The benefits may last several weeks or longer after multiple treatments, but as the disease progresses and the treatment wears off, another cycle of acupuncture treatments will be required to see benefits.

## Are There Risks with Acupuncture?

The risk of complications with acupuncture is limited (human patients have a 7% risk of minor pain or bleeding). Dog owners should be fully aware of these risks and have realistic expectations before selecting this therapy.

# Chiropractic Therapy

**Chiropractic therapy** involves the use of rapid controlled impacts, applied by hand or with a small instrument, to the spine, with the goal of "adjusting" the spinal column and relieving "malalignments." Chiropractors have claimed many uses for these techniques in dogs, but at this time there is no scientific evidence to support these claims. To date, there are no conditions in dogs for which scientific studies support the use of chiropractic treatments.

Some of the most commonly stated reasons for the use of chiropractic involve **lameness** and neck and back problems. Particularly in these cases, chiropractic techniques risk further injury or even death. Patients with these problems may be weakened by cancer, serious spinal disease, or joint disease, and even mild manipulations can cause paralysis, fracture, or severe joint injury.

## Where We Stand

Because of the lack of any proven usefulness, the absence of adequate regulation and certification, and the risks of serious injury, we strongly discourage the use of chiropractic techniques in the treatment of joint disease and osteoarthritis in dogs.

The practice of veterinary chiropractic is generally unregulated. Even though certification is provided by the American Veterinary Chiropractic Association (AVCA), a review of the AVCA directory demonstrates that most so-called veterinary chiropractors are not veterinarians.

Because of the lack of any proven usefulness, the absence of adequate regulation and certification, and the risks of serious injury, we strongly discourage the use of chiropractic techniques in the treatment of joint disease and osteoarthritis in dogs.

# Homeopathy, Holistic, and Herbal Therapy

In **homeopathy**, very small doses of theoretically toxic substances are administered to a patient to boost the immune system, much like a vaccination. Holistic treatment may include numerous alternative therapies and has a central focus on diet. In **herbal therapy,** herbs are used as an alternative to traditional drugs as a way of treating disease. Some herbal remedies, such as devil's claw, phytodolor, and willow bark extract, have been shown to be useful in the relief of pain in human osteoarthritis, but there is no current evidence to support the use of herbal therapy, homeopathy, or holistic medicine in the treatment of joint disease in dogs. Some of these products carry the risk of toxicity or allergic reactions. We recommend that the owners of dogs with joint disease talk to a veterinarian before significantly changing their pet's diet or using any supplements.

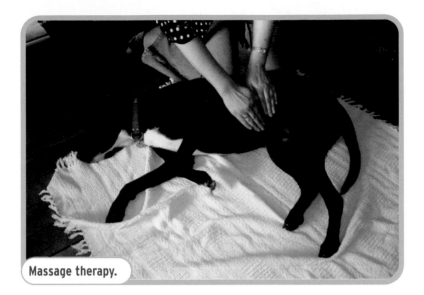

Massage therapy.

# Massage Therapy

Massage therapy may be very effective as a complementary treatment when used by a licensed veterinary physical rehabilitation therapists. Such therapists can train dog owners in simple massage techniques, but because of the risk of severe injury to the spine and legs, we recommend that massage therapy not be administered by anyone other than licensed professionals.

# PART THREE

# Specific Joints and Osteoarthritis

# CHAPTER 12

# OSTEOARTHRITIS OF THE SHOULDER JOINT

Osteoarthritis of the shoulder joint is less common than arthritis in other joints, but arthroscopy is revealing more cases and helping veterinarians understand the causes and determine the best treatment of this problem. In this chapter we discuss the common diseases of the shoulder joint and describe how they are diagnosed and treated.

## Causes

Causes of shoulder arthritis include:

- **Osteochondritis dissecans (OCD)**
- **Ligament and tendon diseases**

224

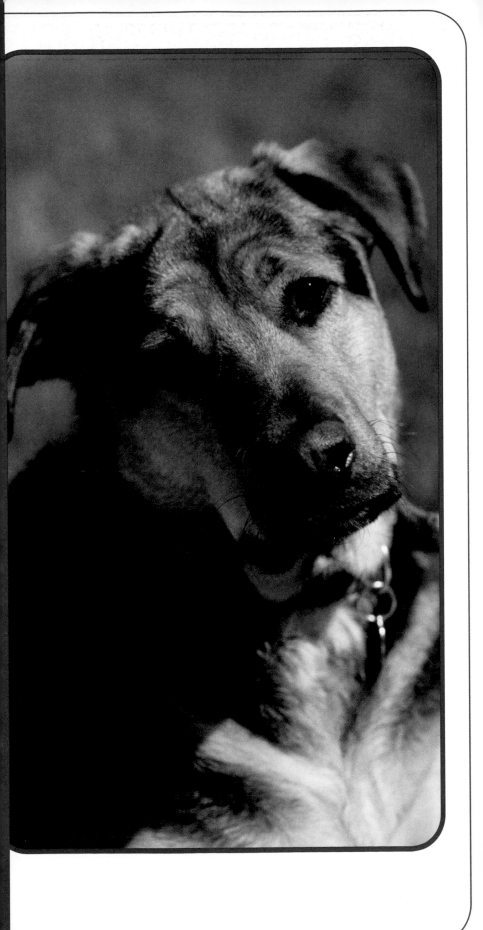

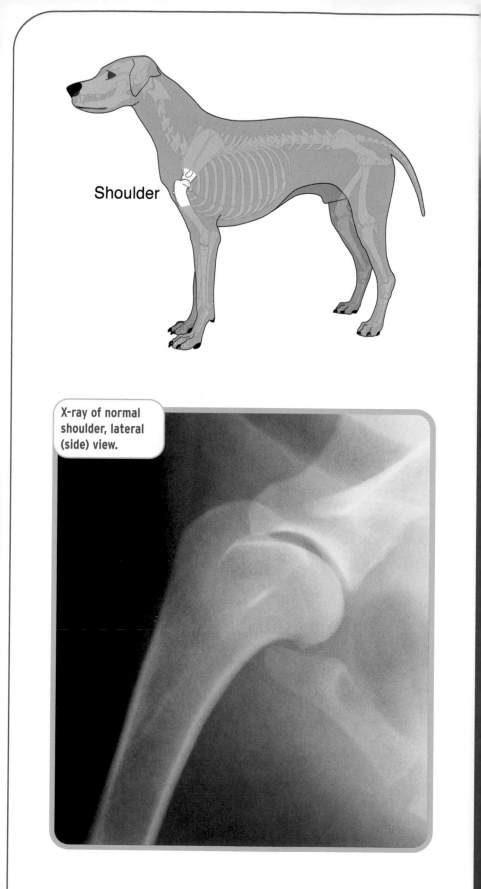

Shoulder

X-ray of normal shoulder, lateral (side) view.

# Osteochondritis Dissecans

OCD of the shoulder joint is probably the leading cause of osteoarthritis in this joint.

OCD of the shoulder is usually found in young dogs ranging from 6 months to 2 years of age. In older dogs that are being examined for shoulder arthritis with arthroscopy, it is often possible to see an old, untreated OCD lesion that is the cause of chronic osteoarthritis.

The clinical sign of shoulder OCD is **lameness** of one or both forelegs. Dogs with shoulder OCD may have trouble getting up and often have some muscle loss and pain when the joint is moved. The diagnosis is usually straightforward because most lesions are easy to see on radiographs (x-rays) of the shoulder joint. The normal curve of the joint surface is interrupted by a flat area representing the abnormal cartilage.

It should be noted that the presence of an OCD-type lesion on an x-ray doesn't mean that there is a flap of cartilage. The x-ray will look the same regardless of whether the thickened cartilage is intact or has become a flap. Only direct observation through arthroscopy or arthrotomy can show whether the lesion is a flap, although in

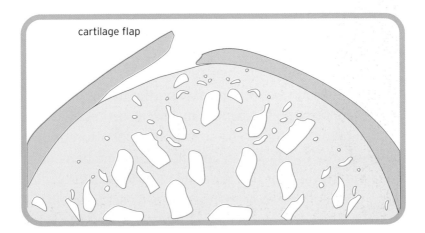
cartilage flap

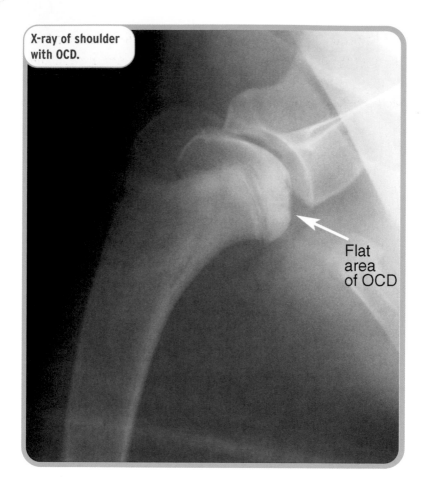

X-ray of shoulder with OCD.

Flat area of OCD

most cases the dog will be in pain only if the cartilage has formed a flap.

Treatment of shoulder OCD should be strongly considered by dog owners. Surgery is usually successful in both the short and the long term; **conservative** (nonsurgical) **management** often means continued limping and may result in severe osteoarthritis later in life.

Surgical treatment involves removing the loose cartilage flap, through either arthroscopy (the use of a "scope" to look into the joint and allow insertion of instruments for treatment) or arthrotomy (open surgery). Removing the cartilage flap lets the underlying bone heal, stops the irritation of the opposing cartilage surface, and keeps the flap from moving into another part of the joint, where it might also cause pain or interference. After the flap is removed, the underlying bed is drilled, "picked," or scraped until it is bleeding. This is done to encourage the defect in the cartilage to heal. The defect will heal not with normal cartilage but with a durable **"fibrocartilage"** that will protect the underlying bone and slow down the osteoarthritis.

The choice between arthrotomy and arthroscopy depends on the surgeon, the price, and personal opinion. Even though no definitive advantages of arthroscopy have been shown, most surgeons agree that it is less invasive, can be performed as quickly as arthrotomy, provides a better view of the joint, and permits treatment that's as good as or better than what can be achieved with arthrotomy.

After surgery for shoulder OCD, it is important to follow your veterinarian's instructions for medical management of osteoarthritis (Chapter 5), including medications and weight control. Fortunately, the outlook for shoulder OCD is generally excellent when it is treated early.

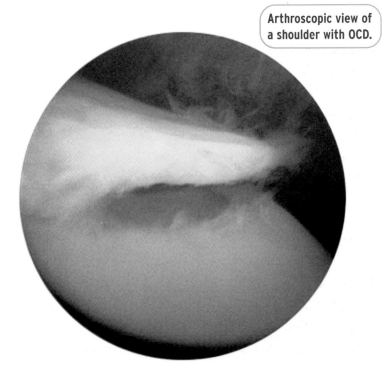

Arthroscopic view of a shoulder with OCD.

# Tendon and Ligament Diseases

The biceps tendon is inside the shoulder joint, so diseases of the tendon can contribute to inflammation of the joint—which can lead to osteoarthritis. Diseases of the biceps tendon can be diagnosed with **ultrasound, magnetic resonance imaging (MRI),** specialized x-ray techniques, or arthroscopy. Rest and medical therapy are often used in mild cases as an alternative to surgery, but if moderate or severe tearing of the ligament is present, surgical treatment is needed. Treatment may be performed as open surgery or by arthroscopy.

Arthroscopic views of a normal *(left)* and torn *(right)* biceps tendon.

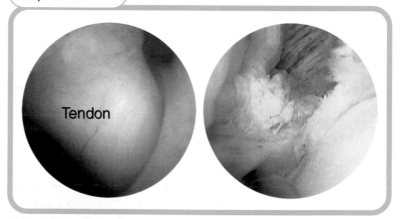

Tendon

Ligaments maintain the stability of joints, and damage to ligaments leads to joint instability and osteoarthritis. Ligament diseases of the shoulder joint are not very well understood but are becoming more commonly recognized through the use of ultrasound, MRI, and, particularly, arthroscopy. Most of the ligaments of the shoulder joint can be seen with the arthroscope, and both arthroscopic and open surgical techniques are being developed to treat these problems.

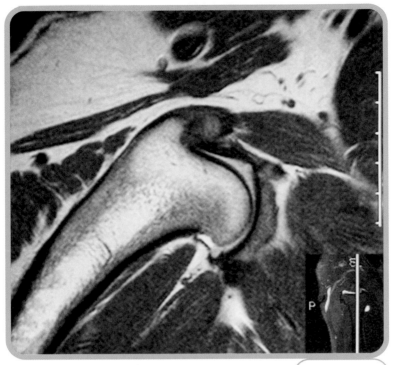

MRI slice of
shoulder joint.

Now let's review the information in this chapter:

- **The most common diseases of the shoulder joint in dogs are osteochondritis dissecans (also known as OCD) and damage of the ligaments and tendons surrounding the joint.**
- **OCD is common in young dogs, and it can be successfully treated with traditional surgery or arthroscopy.**
- **Diseases of the ligaments and tendons around the shoulder (like rotator cuff injuries in people) are not well understood, and they are sometimes difficult to treat.**

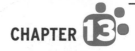

# OSTEOARTHRITIS OF THE ELBOW JOINT

Osteoarthritis of the elbow joint is the most common cause of foreleg lameness in dogs. Many of the arthritic diseases of the elbow are considered forms of developmental elbow malformation (dysplasia). Other injuries may be caused by trauma, but elbow dysplasia is much more common. Elbow dysplasia is a genetic disease that can damage cartilage or bone, starting the process of osteoarthritis. The specific causes of elbow dysplasia are a matter of controversy, as is the best way to treat it. In this chapter we look at these diseases of the elbow joint and the current and future treatments.

## Causes

Common causes of elbow **arthritis** in dogs include:

- Elbow dysplasia
- Fractures
- Luxation

## Elbow Dysplasia

Elbow **dysplasia** refers to a group of congenital diseases of the elbow in dogs, the most common of which are:

- Un-united anconeal process
- Osteochondritis dissecans (OCD)
- Fragmented coronoid process

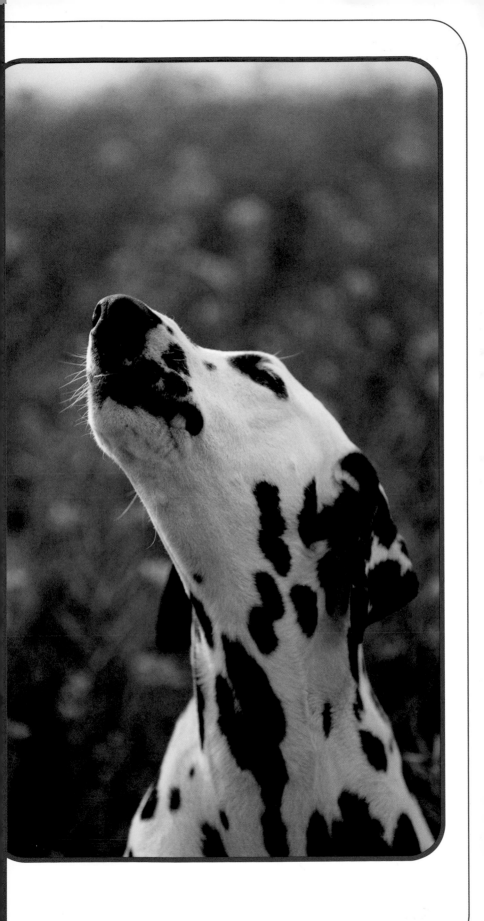

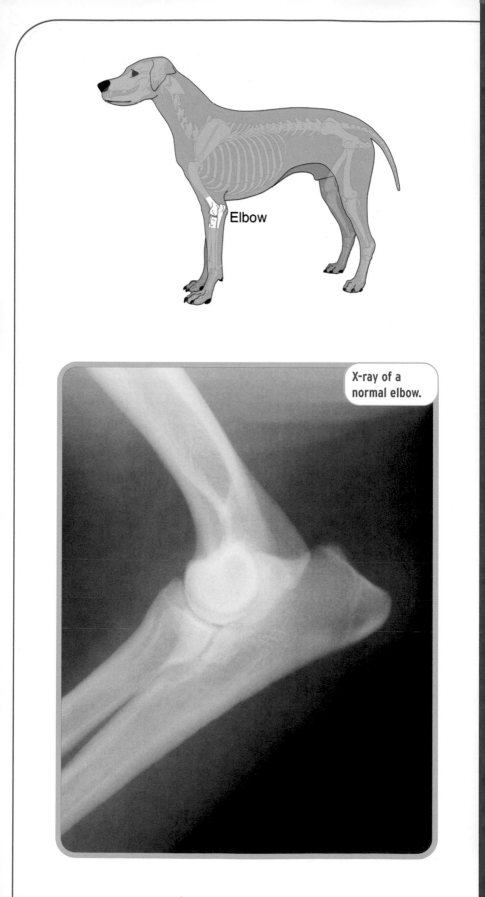

Elbow

X-ray of a normal elbow.

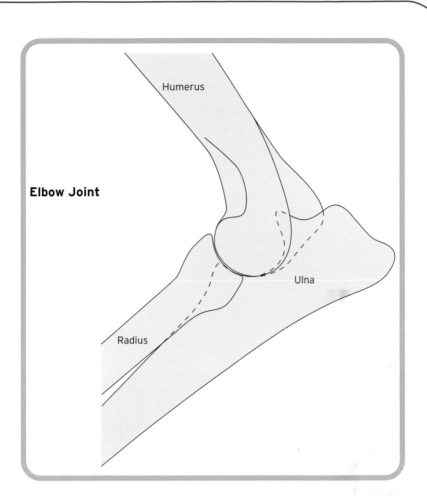

**Elbow Joint**

Humerus

Ulna

Radius

## Un-united Anconeal Process

The anconeal process is a projection of bone at the top end of the ulna (one of the bones of the elbow). Earlier in development, this process is a separate piece of bone. In some dog breeds, especially German Shepherds, the anconeal process may fail to unite with the rest of the ulna during a puppy's growth in the first year of life. This **un-united anconeal process** is then a loose piece of bone within the joint, which contributes to joint instability and inflammation. In many cases, rapid and severe osteoarthritis results. The cause of this problem is still unknown, but it may have something to do with an abnormal rate of growth of the bones of the elbow joint. It is most likely a genetic disease.

Diagnosis of un-united anconeal process is easily made with x-rays in dogs older than 6 months. Treatment remains a matter of controversy, but it will require surgery to either remove or stabilize the unattached bone. The most promising surgical treatment to date involves securing the loose piece of bone with a screw and making a cut **(osteotomy)** in the ulna to release pressure on the surgically attached bit of bone, to encourage healing. The key to successful surgery for un-united anconeal process appears to be early diagnosis, when the osteoarthritis is not yet severe and the body is still able to heal the un-united process to the remainder of the bone.

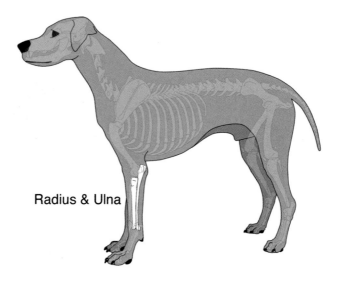

Radius & Ulna

In many cases of un-united anconeal process, the diagnosis comes too late. In these cases, treatment mainly involves aggressive medical management of osteoarthritis. Dogs respond to this osteoarthritis in various ways, but unfortunately, significant loss of joint motion and periodic or chronic pain are common.

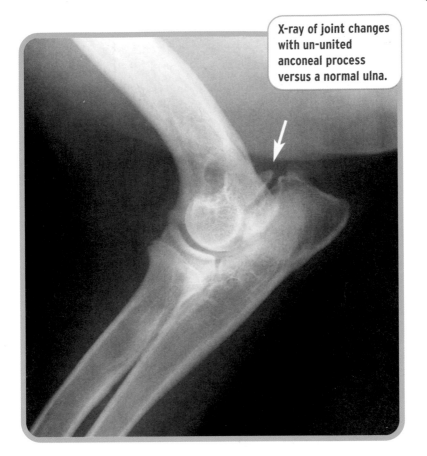

X-ray of joint changes with un-united anconeal process versus a normal ulna.

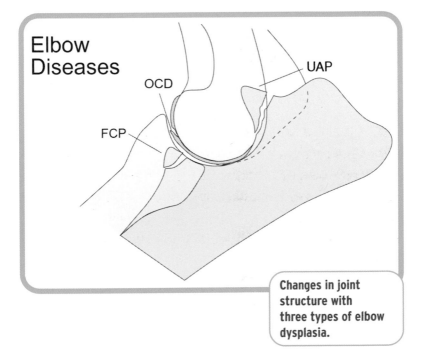

# Elbow Diseases

OCD

UAP

FCP

Changes in joint structure with three types of elbow dysplasia.

# Osteochondritis Dissecans

    OCD of the elbow is usually recognized in young dogs, ranging in age from 6 months to 2 years.

    The clinical sign of elbow OCD is lameness of one or both forelimbs. A dog with this condition may also have difficulty getting up and often has some muscle loss and pain when the elbow joint is moved. The diagnosis requires high-quality radiographs (x-rays) of the elbow joint,

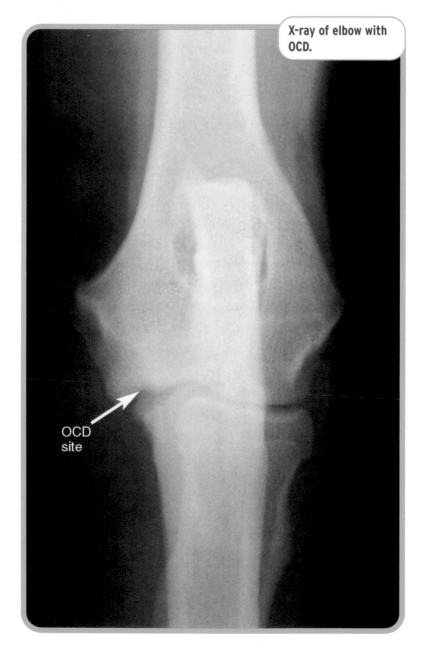

X-ray of elbow with OCD.

OCD site

but even though radiographs can show an old OCD lesion, they cannot show the condition of the remaining cartilage of the joint. So making predictions about the condition based on x-rays is very difficult. In some dogs, the OCD lesion is the only site of cartilage damage in the elbow; in others, extensive full-thickness cartilage loss may already have occurred.

Treatment of elbow OCD involves removing the loose cartilage flap, through either **arthroscopy** (the use of a scope to see into the joint and insert instruments for flap removal) or **arthrotomy** (open surgery). Removal of the cartilage flap may allow the underlying bone to heal with scar tissue, stopping the irritation that occurs when it rubs against the opposing cartilage surface. After the flap is removed, the underlying bed is drilled, "picked," or scraped until it is bleeding, to promote proper healing.

The success of surgical treatment of elbow OCD has been debated, and some veterinarians believe that medical treatment of osteoarthritis provides results similar to those with surgical removal of the flap. Unfortunately, the outlook for elbow OCD is not as good as it is for shoulder OCD. This is probably because OCD of the elbow damages much more of the cartilage surface of the elbow joint than with shoulder OCD. In addition, other forms of elbow

Arthroscopic view of elbow with OCD.

Cartilage Flap

dysplasia may accompany OCD of the elbow, particularly fragmentation of the **medial coronoid process**.

The choice between arthrotomy and arthroscopy depends on the surgeon, the price, and personal opinion. Although no definitive advantages of arthroscopy have been shown, most surgeons agree that it is less invasive, can be performed as quickly as arthrotomy, provides a better view of the joint, and permits therapy as good as or better than what can be done with arthrotomy.

After surgery for elbow OCD, it is important to follow your veterinarian's instructions for medical management of osteoarthritis. Because of the somewhat uncertain outlook, medical treatment of elbow osteoarthritis may be lifelong.

# Fragmented Coronoid Process

**Fragmented coronoid process** (FCP) is the most common form of elbow dysplasia in dogs. In this disease, a fragment of bone and cartilage of one of the bones of the elbow joint (ulna) is broken off. This fragment may be small or large and may stay in place or move about. More important, the rest of the joint may be normal, or there may be additional cartilage damage, including OCD or severe full-thickness cartilage loss.

The cause of FCP is unknown. Common theories include abnormal differences in growth rates between the radius and the ulna—two of the three bones that make up the elbow joint. The elbow joint is one of the most complex joints of the body, and the three bones must fit together precisely to avoid damage to the cartilage and bone. If the elbow bones do not fit perfectly together, the cartilage will wear down and the underlying bone may crack. Poor fit of the bones of the elbow joint is often referred to as **incongruence**. Incongruence is difficult to detect; many veterinarians use x-rays to find it, but the slight incongruence that may lead to FCP is difficult to find on plain x-rays. New techniques using **computed tomography (CT)** scans are being developed to more accurately diagnose incongruence of the elbow in dogs.

## A Hinge Joint

The elbow joint is a hinge joint, and a door hinge is a good comparison. A door hung on a poorly made hinge will begin to sag, and the hinge will start to wear out, with damage to the metal and eventual failure of the hinge.

The treatment of FCP is controversial and complex. In many cases, medical treatment for osteoarthritis is required. Mild FCP may require medical treatment from time to time; severe cases may require continuous intensive therapy.

The simplest form of surgical therapy for FCP is removal of the loose fragment. This may be performed in open surgery or with arthroscopy. Fragment removal alone may significantly improve the quality of life for a dog that has fragments only and no additional cartilage damage; unfortunately, it is impossible to see additional cartilage damage on x-rays or CT scans.

When cartilage damage is seen during **arthroscopy,** the surgeon may perform various techniques to encour-

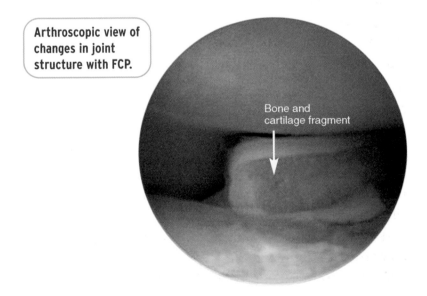

Arthroscopic view of changes in joint structure with FCP.

Bone and cartilage fragment

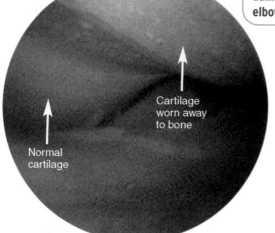

Arthroscopic view of damaged cartilage in elbow.

Normal cartilage

Cartilage worn away to bone

age cartilage healing. These include microfracture and abrasion arthroplasty. These techniques are designed to bring blood supply to the area of damaged cartilage. They may help in some cases but probably will not lead to complete healing of the damaged areas and elimination of the pain of osteoarthritis.

**Osteotomy** is another surgical technique that may be recommended for the treatment of osteoarthritis. Osteotomy involves the cutting of one or more of the bones around a joint to improve the way the joint functions.

The first kind of osteotomy involves cutting the ulna, one of the lower two bones of the elbow. The ulna is cut to allow it to lower or rotate, because some researchers think that elevation of the ulna leads to FCP. Although this procedure has been used for several years, no studies have demonstrated its usefulness. Yet, if elevation of the ulna can be shown to be the cause of FCP, this surgical procedure may have a place in its treatment.

Other osteotomies designed to treat FCP involve cutting the radius and cutting the humerus. Both of these procedures are experimental, and there is little information available to support their effectiveness.

For severe cases of canine elbow dysplasia and osteoarthritis, elbow replacement has recently been developed. Initial reports have been promising, and the effectiveness of elbow replacement in dogs should become more apparent over the next few years as this technique become more widely available.

Now let's review the information in this chapter:

- **The most common causes of osteoarthritis of the elbow are elbow dysplasia, luxation, and fracture.**
- **Elbow dysplasia includes three diseases: ununited anconeal process, fragmentation of the coronoid process, and osteochondritis dissecans, or OCD.**
- **Elbow dysplasia may be associated with mild or severe osteoarthritis, so the veterinarian cannot give a prognosis until the joint has been inspected.**
- **Arthroscopy is an excellent way to see and operate in the dog's elbow joint.**
- **Artificial replacements for the elbow are being developed and tested in clinics around the world.**

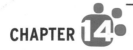

# OSTEOARTHRITIS OF THE CARPAL JOINT (WRIST)

Osteoarthritis and joint disease of the carpus, or wrist, in the dog are fairly common. The most common causes are trauma in active dogs and joint disease involving the immune system in smaller dogs. Some of these diseases are challenging to treat, but the carpus can be permanently fused, with excellent results. In this chapter we discuss the common diseases of the carpus and how these diseases are diagnosed and treated.

## Causes

The two most common causes of osteoarthritis of the carpus are:

- Trauma
- Immune-mediated joint disease

## Trauma

Trauma to the **carpus** is unusual but does occur in automobile accidents and falls. In most cases, the **ligaments** surrounding the joint are torn, causing joint instability and osteoarthritis. Therapy for these injuries depends on the structures that have been damaged. In most cases, surgery is required to stabilize the joint and is important in minimizing osteoarthritis.

When severe osteoarthritis of the carpus does occur, the joint can be fused, with an outstanding outcome. Fusion of a joint is referred to as arthrodesis. When performed successfully on the carpus, it eliminates os-

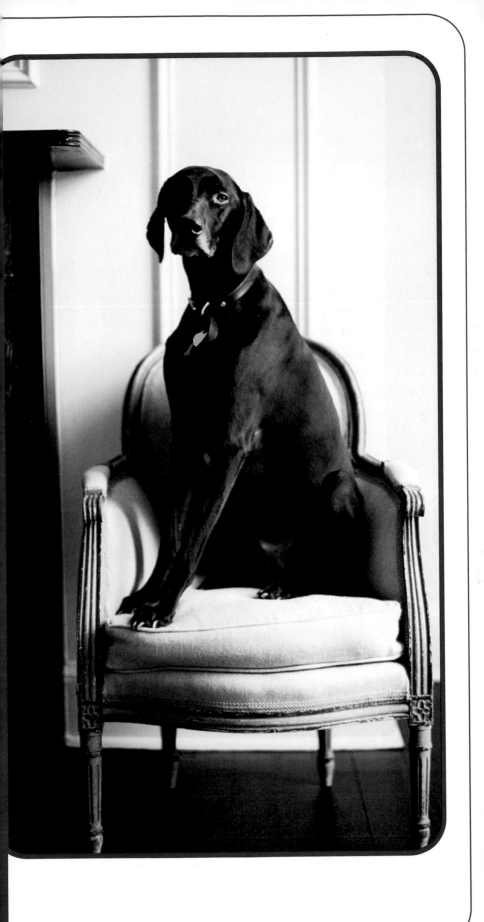

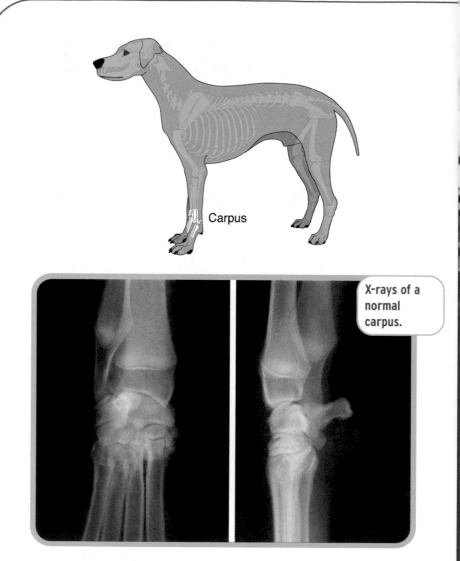

Carpus

X-rays of a normal carpus.

teoarthritis pain permanently. In addition, once the fusion has healed, the dog can return to full activity, and in most cases it is hard to tell that the dog ever had the procedure. The dog will use the leg normally in running, jumping, and all other activities.

# Immune-Mediated Joint Disease

When a dog has immune-mediated joint disease, it is often most easily recognized in the carpus. The swelling of this joint is easily seen and felt. Small dogs are often affected, although any dog can have immune-mediated joint disease.

X-rays of a normal carpus and hyperextension of the carpus due to immune-mediated joint disease or trauma.

Diagnostics should include **joint fluid** analysis and evaluation of the other organs of the body for a primary cause. Other diseases such as cancer and gastrointestinal diseases may cause immune-mediated joint disease; however, in most cases no other diseases are found. Treatment usually includes **steroids;** the outlook is good to excellent.

Now let's review the information in this chapter:

- **Trauma and joint disease involving the immune system are the most common causes of osteoarthritis of the carpus in dogs.**
- **Most dogs with trauma to the carpus have fallen or jumped, severely straining the carpus. This is a serious injury, but fusion (arthrodesis) of the carpus usually has outstanding results.**
- **Immune joint diseases (similar to rheumatoid arthritis or lupus in people) are more common in smaller dogs and in smaller joints, such as the carpus.**
- **Immune joint disease often causes the joints to break down or collapse.**
- **Your veterinarian can diagnose immune joint disease by sampling the fluid in the joint. Steroids are usually prescribed.**
- **Severe collapse of the carpus caused by immune joint disease can be treated with arthrodesis.**

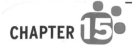

# OSTEOARTHRITIS OF THE HIP JOINT

The hip joint is the most common location of osteoarthritis in dogs because of the high incidence of hip dysplasia. Luxations (dislocations) and fractures of the hip can also cause osteoarthritis, but these injuries are much less common than hip dysplasia. Fortunately, there are many surgical and medical treatments for osteoarthritis of the hip. In this chapter we discuss the causes and signs of osteoarthritis of the hip and the many treatments available.

## Causes

The most common causes of osteoarthritis of the hip are:

- Hip dysplasia
- Hip luxation

## Hip Dysplasia

Hip dysplasia is likely the best known and most common cause of **arthritis** in dogs. Dysplasia technically means "abnormal development." Hip dysplasia is therefore the abnormal development of the hip joint. Hip dysplasia is a genetic disease that can be made worse but is not caused by activity or diet. The specific abnormalities of hip joint development that cause hip dysplasia are not known, but they likely include laxity (looseness) and abnormal shape of the bones that make up the joint. The bones of the hip joint include the femur (specifically the femoral head) and the "bony pelvis" (specifically the acetabulum). The two bones are held together by a **ligament,** a joint capsule, and the muscles of the hip.

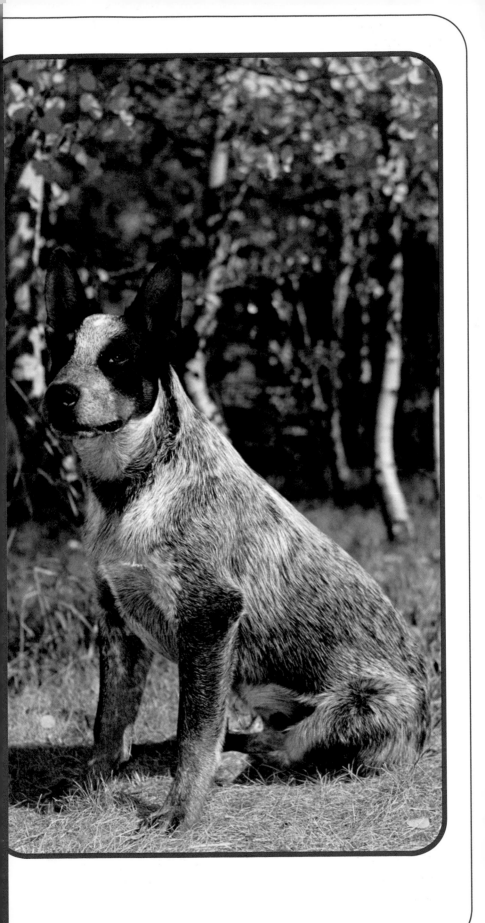

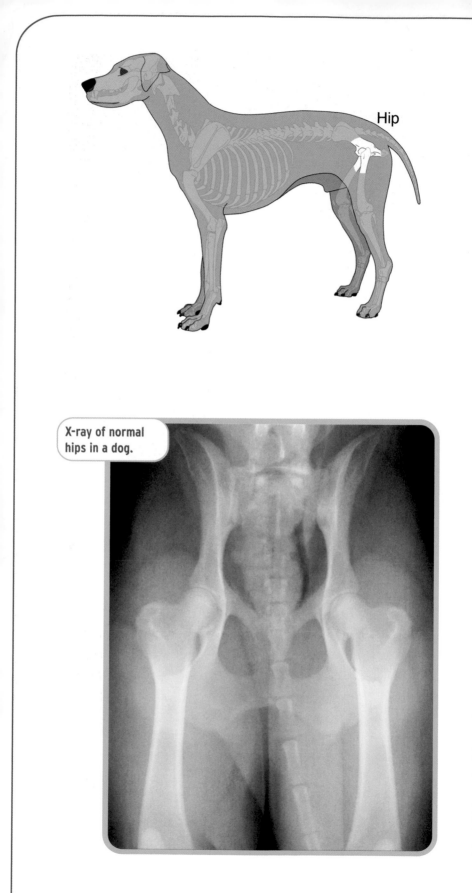

Hip

X-ray of normal hips in a dog.

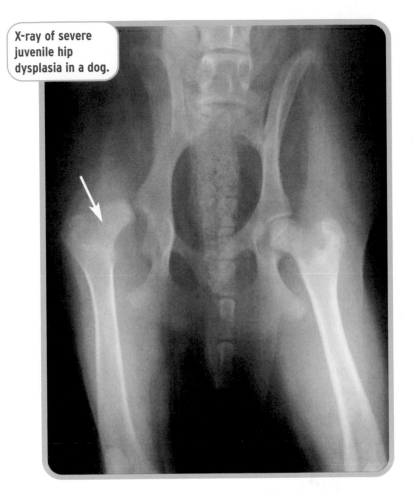

X-ray of severe juvenile hip dysplasia in a dog.

In juvenile dogs (younger than 18 months of age), when the bones of the hip are improperly shaped, the ball-and-socket joint becomes loose, which may cause damage to the cartilage of the joint and then osteoarthritis. The ball (femoral head) may begin to move out of the socket (acetabulum) as the animal walks or runs. This is referred to as subluxation. In the worst cases, the femoral head may come completely out of the acetabulum (luxation). In most cases, however, there is only subluxation, which leads to destruction of the cartilage and malformation of the joint as the dog matures.

In young dogs, the pain of hip dysplasia comes mainly from the subluxation. This abnormal movement of the joint causes tension on the soft tissues around the joint, resulting in great pain.

# The Two Phases of Hip Dysplasia

Hip dysplasia is a two-phase disease with two different causes of pain. The first cause is subluxation of the hip joint, which stretches and tears the soft tissues around the joint. This pain eases as the joint "scars down" and tightens with age. The second and later cause of pain is osteoarthritis due to damage to the cartilage and the misshapen ball and socket.

In most cases, as the dog matures, the pain of subluxation eases as the soft tissues around the joint "scar down" and the subluxation disappears. Young adult dogs may show significant decrease in clinical signs, even without treatment.

The second stage of hip dysplasia is the arthritic stage. Although the joint is no longer loose or subluxating, the joint is not normally formed. It is no longer a perfect ball and socket, as it is in a normal dog. Usually the ball and socket are flattened. This abnormal shape contributes to the damage to cartilage that occurred during the juvenile stage, to further the process of osteoarthritis and subsequent pain.

Many dogs with hip dysplasia never show a sign of pain during their entire lifetime. A few dogs will have transient signs of pain caused by the subluxation but never show pain due to arthritis; still others will improve after the early stage and not show signs of arthritis for many months or years. In a large population of dogs, the juvenile stage will not be seen, but they will demonstrate signs of hip arthritis during their middle or later years. In the most severe cases, the dog will have uninterrupted pain from the juvenile stage to the arthritic stage.

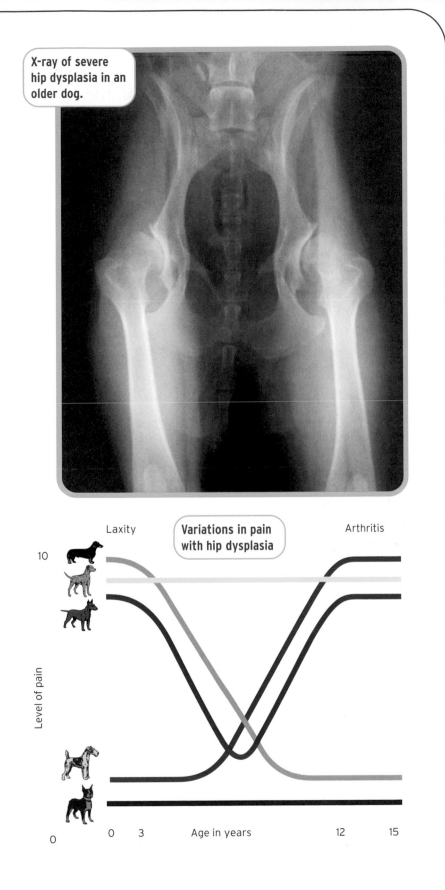

X-ray of severe hip dysplasia in an older dog.

Variations in pain with hip dysplasia

Laxity

Arthritis

Level of pain

10

0

0   3          Age in years          12    15

Diagnosis of hip dysplasia is based mainly on **palpation** and x-rays. Palpation (examination and manipulation by hand) often reveals muscle loss and pain on extension of the hip joint. In a young dog, the veterinarian may be able to feel the joint subluxation, particularly if the dog is sedated or anesthetized. These findings help the doctor judge the severity and stage of the dysplasia.

There are many techniques for getting x-rays of the hips to look for hip dysplasia. The most basic technique is to lay the dog on its back with the legs extended. An x-ray obtained using this technique is often referred to as the OFA view because it is the view used by the Orthopedic Foundation for Animals (OFA) to grade the severity of the disease in dogs older than 2 years. It is the most common view used to evaluate the severity of osteoarthritis and the degree of subluxation, but its accuracy in determining subluxation has been questioned. A technique specifically designed to evaluate joint laxity as the cause of subluxation is the PennHip method (PennHip stands for the University of Pennsylvania Hip Improvement Program). For the PennHip view, gentle force is applied to determine the severity of subluxation. Both the PennHip and the OFA organizations use these views to predict osteoarthritis in dogs later in life and to help make recommendations for breeders with regard to hip dysplasia. These views are also used by veterinarians and surgeons to help make recommendations about the best treatment for individual dogs.

Therapy for hip dysplasia can be separated into medical and surgical treatments. Medical treatment is similar for younger and for older dogs and involves analgesics, weight control, nutritional supplements, and exercise management or physical therapy.

Surgical treatment for hip dysplasia differs from dog to dog, depending on age. The basic categories of these surgical procedures are:

- **Modification of the joint**
- **Removal of the joint**
- **Replacement of the joint**

# Modification of the Joint by Triple Pelvic Osteotomy or Juvenile Pubic Symphysiodesis

In the young growing patient without significant osteoarthritis, the surgeon may recommend trying to improve the joint and stop the subluxation. This procedure involves twisting the socket (acetabulum) by cutting and rotating the bone. This results in decreased subluxation and therefore less pain. It may also dramatically decrease the progression of arthritis later in life. In very young dogs, this may be achieved with a technique called juvenile pubic symphysiodesis, but for the most benefit, the hip dysplasia must be diagnosed before the dog is 20 weeks of age. In older dogs, modification of the joint is accomplished in a surgical procedure called triple pelvic **osteotomy** (TPO). In this procedure, the pelvis is cut in three places to permit rotation of the acetabulum, to stop the femoral head from subluxating. The success of this procedure depends mainly on careful patient selection. The deciding factors include:

- **Age**
- **Severity of subluxation**
- **Severity of osteoarthritis**
- **Function of the dog**

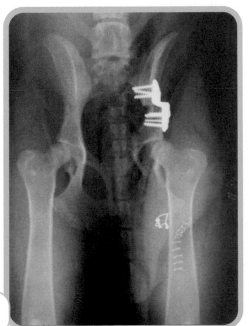

X-ray of the hip in a dog after TPO.

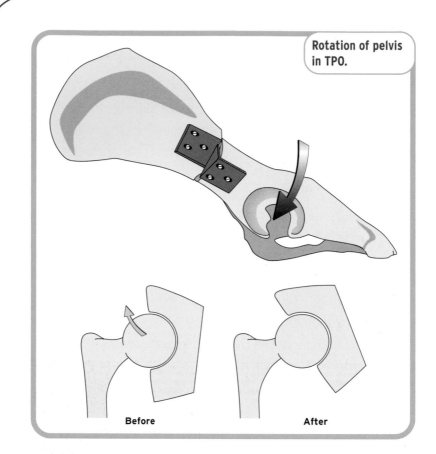

Rotation of pelvis in TPO.

Before                    After

## Removal of the Joint by Femoral Head Ostectomy

In severe cases of hip dysplasia with luxation or severe arthritis, removal of the joint may be chosen. This procedure is called a femoral head (and neck) **ostectomy** (FHO). In this procedure, the ball of the ball and socket is removed so that the femur and the pelvic bone no longer make contact. The femur and the leg are supported by the strong muscles surrounding the hip joint, making the hind leg work like the foreleg does—the foreleg has no joint connecting it to the spine.

The success of the FHO procedure depends mostly on the size of the dog and the strength of the muscles around the hip. Smaller dogs tend to have better outcomes than larger dogs, but the outcome in larger dogs can be significantly improved by keeping body weight low and encouraging activities that strengthen the muscles around the hip.

The success of an FHO should not be judged for several months after surgery, because dogs tend to improve over time as the hip adjusts by forming scar tissue and strengthening the muscles. The use of physical rehabilitation may dramatically improve the outcome of FHO in dogs.

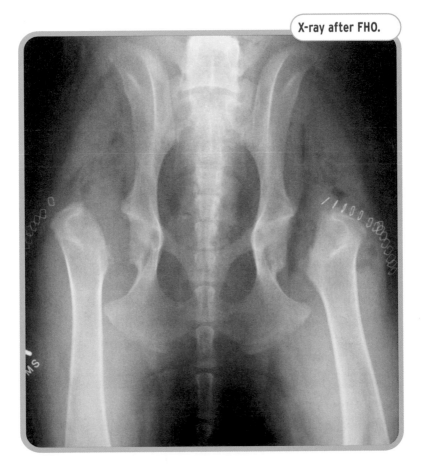

X-ray after FHO.

# Replacement of the Joint by Total Hip Replacement

In severe cases of hip dysplasia, the surgeon may recommend total hip replacement (THR). This procedure involves replacing both the femoral head and the acetabulum (the ball and socket) with high-grade implants similar to those used in people. These implants are available in both cemented and noncemented varieties. Both techniques appear to give outstanding results in 80% to 90% of cases, but complications can be expensive and often require an FHO. The main limitation for use of these techniques is their expense.

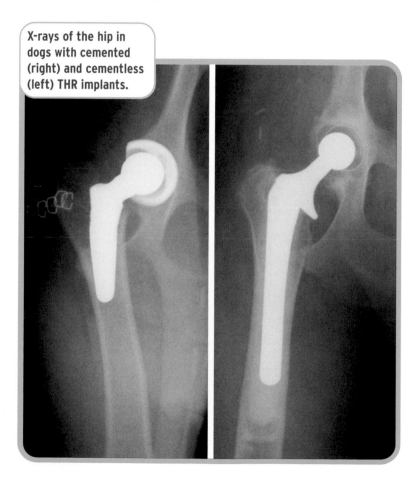

X-rays of the hip in dogs with cemented (right) and cementless (left) THR implants.

Now let's review the information in this chapter:

- **Hip dysplasia is the best known and most common cause of osteoarthritis of the hip joint in dogs.**
- **Hip dysplasia, a genetic disease, can be made worse but is not caused by activity or diet.**
- **Hip dysplasia in young dogs causes pain because it stretches and tears soft tissues.**
- **Hip dysplasia in older dogs causes pain because of the osteoarthritis that results.**
- **Weight control, moderate exercise, and anti-inflammatory medications are the basic methods used to treat hip dysplasia and osteoarthritis.**
- **Surgery for hip dysplasia in young dogs includes triple pelvic osteotomy, femoral head and neck ostectomy, and, in very young dogs, juvenile pubic symphysiodesis.**
- **In mature dogs, surgery includes femoral head and neck ostectomy and total hip replacement.**

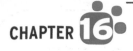

# OSTEOARTHRITIS OF THE KNEE JOINT

Osteoarthritis of the knee is common in dogs. Rupture of a ligament called the cranial cruciate ligament is the usual cause. Surgery to repair a ruptured cruciate ligament is the most common orthopedic procedure in dogs. Rupture of the cruciate ligament is almost always treated with surgery, but the cause of this disease and the best way to treat it are matters of controversy. For this reason it is important that owners of dogs with cruciate ligament tears understand the basics of their surgical options. In this chapter we look at the diagnosis and treatment of cruciate ligament rupture in the dog, plus other diseases of the knee joint.

## Causes

The most common causes of osteoarthritis of the knee are:

- Cranial cruciate ligament rupture
- Patellar luxation
- Trauma
- Osteochondritis dissecans (OCD)
- Immune-mediated joint disease

## Cranial Cruciate Ligament Rupture

Cranial cruciate ligament rupture (CCLR) is the most common orthopedic injury in dogs. The cranial cruciate ligament is one of several ligaments in the knee that maintain the stability of the joint. In people, the same lig-

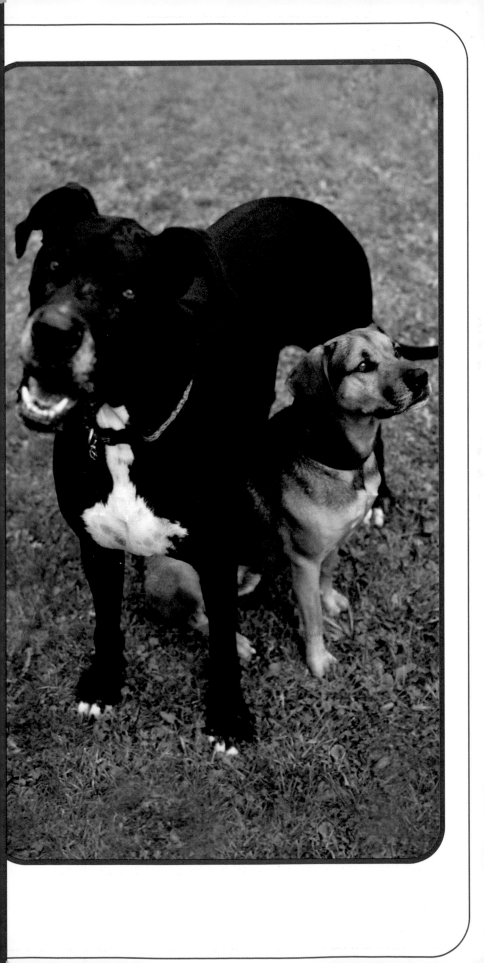

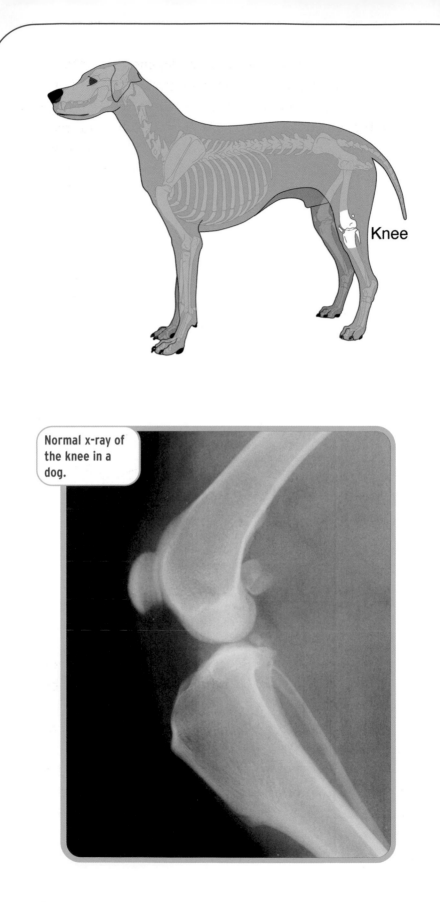

Knee

Normal x-ray of the knee in a dog.

ament is called the anterior cruciate ligament. In both dogs and humans, the ligament may stretch or tear, leading to pain and osteoarthritis. CCLR can also lead to damage to the menisci in the knee. The menisci are two small cushions of **fibrocartilage** that sit between the bones of the knee. CCLR can make the menisci vulnerable to tearing, which is quite painful.

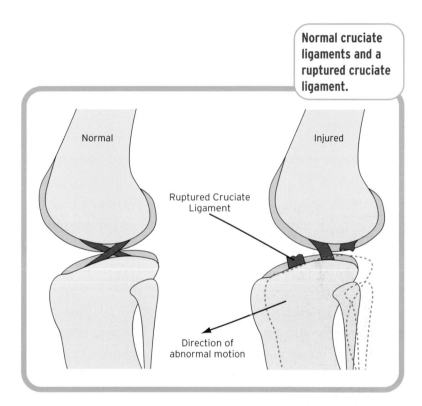

Normal cruciate ligaments and a ruptured cruciate ligament.

Normal

Injured

Ruptured Cruciate Ligament

Direction of abnormal motion

The cause of CCLR is unknown. In people, this common injury is usually associated with trauma from athletic activities such as skiing; however, its occurrence in dogs suggests an underlying abnormality such as **dysplasia** or inflammatory or vascular disease.

The signs of CCLR vary, but they include acute onset of **lameness** followed by mild improvement but continued lameness, or moderately progressive lameness particularly associated with exercise or with getting up after resting.

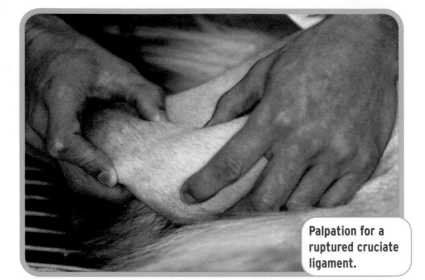

Palpation for a ruptured cruciate ligament.

CCLR is first diagnosed by **palpation** (examination and manipulation by hand). In a dog with a complete rupture, the veterinarian will be able to feel the instability that results. In dogs with stretching or partial tearing, there may be no instability at all, but your veterinarian may suspect CCLR after finding a firm swelling of the knee and seeing that the dog has pain when the joint is moved.

X-rays are routinely taken in dogs with CCLR, but this disease cannot be diagnosed on x-rays because the ligament does not appear. Changes on x-rays with CCLR are identical to those with most diseases that affect the knee joint, although the x-rays may be helpful in judging the severity of osteoarthritis and ruling out other diseases. **MRI (magnetic resonance imaging)** may also be used to diagnose CCLR and damage to the meniscus, but in most cases this study is not necessary or is unavailable. MRI is also expensive and requires general anesthesia in dogs.

CCLR may be diagnosed by arthroscopy before surgical treatment of the ligament rupture. **Arthroscopy** may also be used to see into the joint for "cleaning out" and for treating meniscal injuries with a smaller incision than

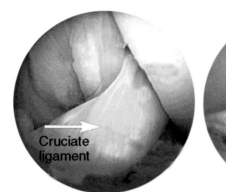

Arthroscopic views of a normal *(left)* and ruptured *(right)* cruciate ligament in a dog.

Cruciate ligament

what traditional surgery would involve. Purely arthroscopic treatments of CCLR are available but are not in widespread use, mainly because of concerns about effectiveness. In this way, the treatment of CCLR in dogs differs dramatically from that in people.

## Treatment of CCLR

Many treatments for CCLR are available, and there is widespread debate and disagreement about the usefulness of these treatments. Surgery is often recommended for medium to large dogs. In small dogs it is possible for the knee to improve in stability without surgery as the body lays down scar tissue around the joint. In most cases, this is best achieved with several weeks to 2 months of strict rest, so that healing can occur without being interrupted by the forces of vigorous activity. Many small dogs, however, will heal without surgery. Treatment by rest alone may be attempted in any size dog, but in larger and more active dogs, adequate stabilization of the knee will usually not be achieved, and the pain and lameness will continue.

More traditional surgical treatments of CCLR involve replacing of the ligament with either a natural or a synthetic material. In these procedures, natural fibrous tissue, nylon suture, or wire is used to stabilize the knee. These procedures have been used for more than half a century, and the results are good to excellent in many cases. The outcome of these procedures may be improved with physical therapy. The main concern with these procedures is that the stabilizing material can stretch or break, after which the knee is stabilized by scar tissue. This may lead to a decrease in the **range of motion** of the joint and allow some progression of osteoarthritis.

Another widely used technique in treatment of CCLR is the tibial plateau leveling ostotomy (TPLO). In this technique, the lower bone of the joint (the tibia) is cut and ro-

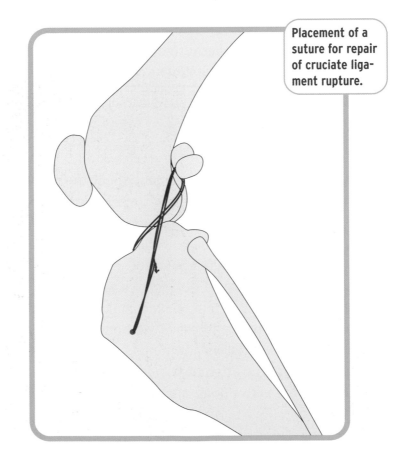

Placement of a suture for repair of cruciate ligament rupture.

tated to eliminate the abnormal motion of the knee during normal activity. The advantage of this procedure is that it does not rely on materials that can stretch or break to stabilize the knee. Disadvantages and concerns include the necessity of cutting bone, the mechanical alterations of the knee, and the higher cost of the procedure. TPLO may be better especially in larger dogs, because their heavier body weight puts more force through the knee, with a greater chance of stretching materials used in traditional repair methods. Although specific advantages of TPLO over traditional methods have yet to be demonstrated, the technique has gained widespread acceptance because of reports of improved results, especially in larger dogs. A new technique is tibial tuberosity advancement (TTA). This procedure is similar to TPLO in that it does not rely on a replacement of the ligament. Because this is a new technique, its success rate is difficult to judge at present.

X-ray of the knee after TPLO for repair of cruciate ligament rupture.

## CCLR and Osteoarthritis

Pain associated with CCLR may be caused by joint instability, damage to the meniscus, or osteoarthritis. There are no complete conclusions about how well each of the surgical methods just described slows or stops the osteoarthritis, but it is accepted that eliminating the joint instability is important in protecting the menisci and slowing the process of osteoarthritis.

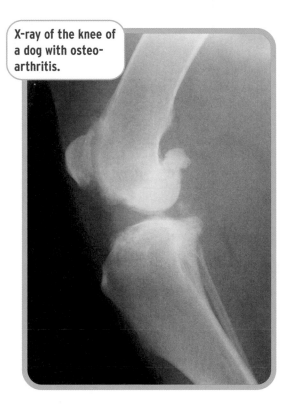

X-ray of the knee of a dog with osteoarthritis.

In mild or early cases of CCLR, medical management of the osteoarthritis after surgery is usually unnecessary, but in more severe cases, medical management may be combined with surgical treatment to eliminate lameness.

# Patellar Luxation

Patellar luxation is a displacement of the patella (kneecap) to the side of the joint. This is most often a congenital disease that is due to poor alignment of the bones and joints of the hind leg. Most commonly there is bowing and/or twisting of the bones above and below the knee. This causes the patella to pop out of the groove in which it is supposed to sit. In mild cases the patella may be in place most of the time and pop out of place from time to time. With increasing severity, the patella is out of alignment more of the time, and in the most severe cases, the patella is out of place all of the time and cannot be pushed into proper alignment.

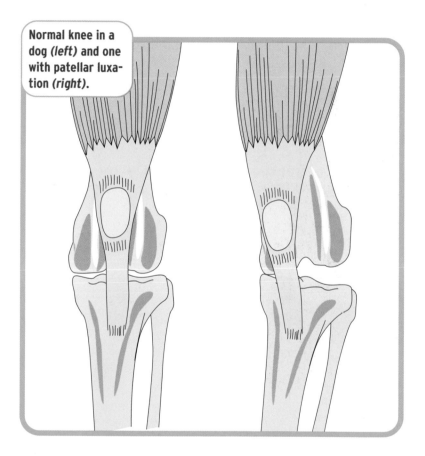

Normal knee in a dog *(left)* and one with patellar luxation *(right)*.

The main clinical sign of patellar luxation is an intermittent hopping on the limb when the patella pops out of alignment. Often the patella pops back in on its own, at which time the dog usually walks normally.

Much of the lameness of patellar luxation is caused by the mechanical insufficiency and soft tissue pain when the patella is out of alignment, but the chronic slippage of the patella does cause cartilage wear and can contribute to osteoarthritis, especially in larger dogs. Correction of the luxation is recommended when the frequency of lameness is significantly affecting the dog's quality of life and function.

Surgical correction of patellar luxation is a routine procedure and highly successful in most cases. In more severe cases, several repair procedures may be required, because the scar tissue that forms during the healing process may pull the patella back out of alignment. The basic procedures that are performed during surgery for patellar luxation include:

- **Soft tissue release in the direction of luxation**
- **Soft tissue tightening (imbrication) opposite the direction of luxation**
- **Deepening the groove where the patella normally rides**
- **Relocation (transposition) of the tibial crest to realign the patella**

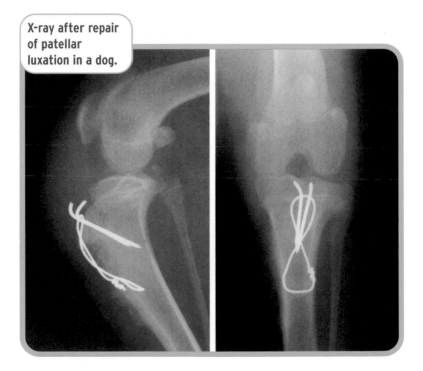

X-ray after repair of patellar luxation in a dog.

Two other procedures that have been described are transposition of the rectus femoris, a muscle that is at the origin of the patellar mechanism, and placement of an "anti-rotation" suture. In the second procedure, a suture is tied between the bones of the knee to rotate them into alignment.

In more severe cases, when the specific malformation of the bone can be identified, it may be necessary to cut the tibia or the femur to correct the underlying bone abnormality that causes the poor alignment of the joint. This method of surgical correction is a little more invasive and requires first cutting and then repair of the bone with a bone plate and screws.

The outlook after correction of patellar luxation is good to excellent, except in severe cases, when several surgical repair procedures may be required to keep the patella in place. Patellar luxation is most common in toy breed dogs. After the correction, osteoarthritis is rarely a problem. This is true of most large dogs with patellar luxation as well, although early surgery is recommended to reduce the severity and slow the progression of osteoarthritis.

# Osteochondritis Dissecans

Osteochondritis dissecans (OCD) of the knee is usually recognized in dogs ranging in age from 6 months to 2 years.

The clinical sign of knee OCD is lameness of one or both hind legs. A dog with OCD may also have difficulty getting up and often has some muscle loss and pain when the knee joint is moved. The diagnosis requires high-quality x-rays of the knee joint.

Treatment of knee OCD involves removing the loose cartilage flap, through either arthroscopy (the use of an endoscope to look into the joint and to insert instruments for flap removal) or arthrotomy (open surgery). Removal of the cartilage flap may help the underlying bone heal and stop the irritation of the opposing cartilage surface. After the flap is removed, the underlying bed is drilled, "picked," or scraped until it is bleeding. This is done to have the bone heal as well as possible. The success of surgical treatment of knee OCD has been debated, and some veterinarians believe that medical treatment provides results similar to those with surgical removal of the flap. Unfortunately, the outlook for knee OCD is not as good as it is for shoulder OCD, probably because OCD of the knee damages a major weight-bearing area of the joint.

The choice between arthrotomy and arthroscopy depends on the surgeon, the price, and personal opinion. Although no definitive advantages of arthroscopy have been demonstrated, most surgeons agree that it is less invasive, can be performed as quickly as arthrotomy, provides a better view of the joint, and permits therapy as good as or better than what can be done in an arthrotomy.

After surgery for knee OCD, it is important to follow your veterinarian's instructions for medical management of osteoarthritis (Chapter 5), including medications and

Arthroscopic view of knee OCD.

Cartilage flap

weight control. Because of the somewhat uncertain outlook, medical treatment of osteoarthritis of the knee may be necessary from time to time or for the life of the dog.

# Immune-Mediated Joint Disease

The knee joint may have immune-mediated joint disease similar to that in other joints. There is also a specific type of immune-mediated joint disease that affects the knee joint (lymphocytic-plasmacytic arthritis).

Now let's review the information in this chapter:

- **Common diseases of the knee joint in dogs include rupture of the cruciate ligament, luxation (dislocation) of the knee cap (patella), and osteochondritis dissecans, or OCD.**
- **In most dogs, the cruciate ligament doesn't rupture because of trauma, but the underlying cause is not understood very well.**
- **Partial tearing of the cruciate ligament is common. A dog with such a tear may experience minor lameness for long periods, and the cause of lameness may be difficult to diagnose.**
- **Rupture of the cruciate ligament usually leads to osteoarthritis; it can also cause damage to the meniscus (two small cartilage cushions in the joint).**
- **Dogs with cruciate ruptures often undergo suture stabilization or tibial plateau leveling osteotomy (TPLO).**
- **Luxation of the kneecap (patellar luxation) is common in small-breed dogs but also occurs in large-breed dogs.**
- **Surgery to treat luxation of the kneecap is usually successful, but severe luxation may be much more difficult to cure.**

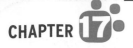

# OSTEOARTHRITIS OF THE HOCK

Osteoarthritis and joint disease of the hock (back ankle) in dogs are common. Most cases are caused by OCD or when a dog is hit by a car. Immune joint disease is a problem in smaller dogs. Although some of these diseases are challenging to treat, the hock can be permanently fused with excellent results. In this chapter we discuss the common diseases of the hock and describe how these diseases are diagnosed and treated.

## Causes

The most common causes of osteoarthritis of the hind leg are:

- Osteochondritis dissecans (OCD)
- Trauma
- Immune-mediated joint disease

## Osteochondritis Dissecans

OCD of the hock is usually recognized in juvenile dogs ranging in age from 6 months to 2 years.

The clinical sign of hock OCD is lameness of one or both hind legs. A dog with OCD may also have difficulty getting up and will often have some muscle loss and pain when the hock joint is manipulated. The diagnosis requires high-quality radiographs (x-rays) of the hock joint.

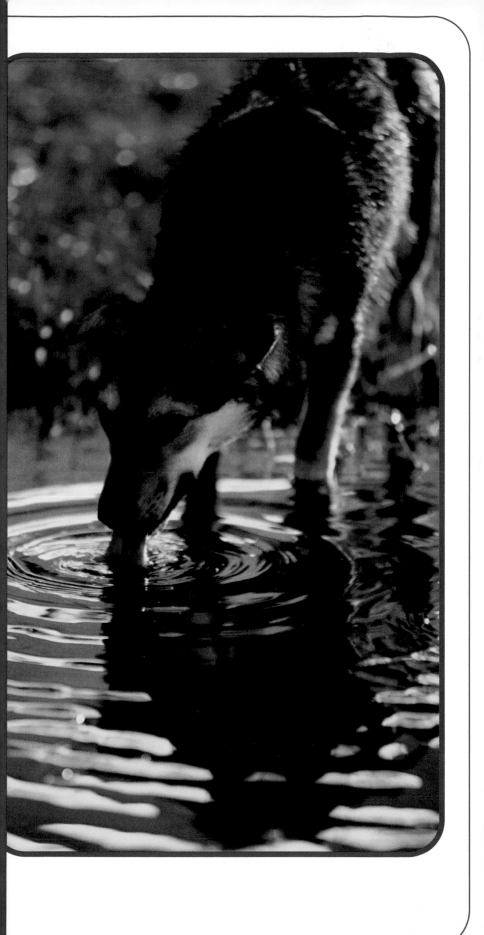

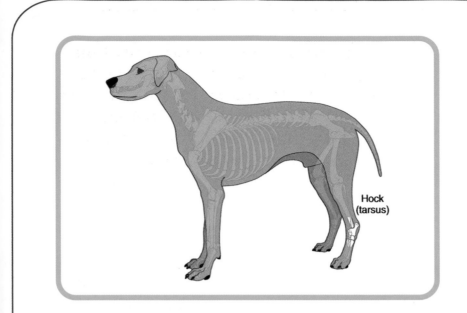

Hock
(tarsus)

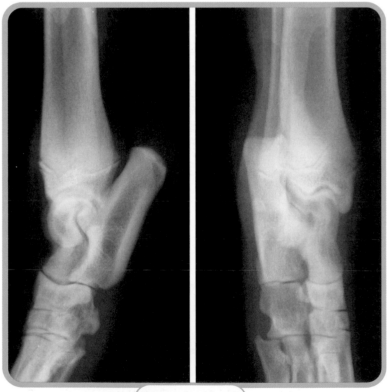

X-rays of a normal hock.

Treatment of hock OCD involves removal of the loose cartilage flap, through either arthroscopy (the use of a endoscope to look into the joint and to insert instruments for flap removal) or arthrotomy (open surgery). Removal of the cartilage flap helps the underlying bone heal and stops the irritation of the opposing cartilage surface. After the flap is removed, the underlying bed is drilled, "picked," or scraped until it is bleeding. This is done to have the bone heal as well as possible. The success of surgical treatment of hock OCD has been debated, and some veterinarians believe that medical management of osteoarthritis provides results similar to those achieved with surgical removal of the flap. Unfortunately, the outlook for hock OCD is not as good as it is for shoulder OCD. This is likely because OCD of the hock damages a major-weight bearing area of the joint.

The choice between arthrotomy and arthroscopy depends on the surgeon, the price, and personal opinion. Although no definitive advantages of arthroscopy have been demonstrated, most surgeons agree that it is less invasive, can be performed as quickly as arthrotomy, provides a better view of the joint, and permits therapy as good as or better than what can be done in an arthrotomy.

After surgery for hock OCD, it is important to follow your veterinarian's instructions for medical management of osteoarthritis (Chapter 5), including medications and weight control. Because of the uncertain outcome, medical management for osteoarthritis of the hock may be necessary from time to time or for the life of the dog. If OCD of the hock results in severe osteoarthritis, surgical fusion (arthrodesis) of the hock joint can be performed for excellent function and complete elimination of pain.

# Immune-Mediated Joint Disease

**Immune-mediated joint disease** often involves the hock because of the large number of small joints that make up this joint. Small dogs are often affected, although any dog may have immune-mediated joint disease.

Diagnostics should include **joint fluid** analysis and evaluation of the rest of the body for a primary cause. Treatment usually includes **steroids,** and the outlook is good to excellent.

# Trauma

Trauma such as being struck by an automobile may result in a fracture or dislocation of the hock joint. Most of these injuries require surgery to repair the fracture or stabilize the joint. In severe cases, fusion (arthrodesis) of the hock joint may be recommended. As previously mentioned, fusion of the hock joint should result in excellent function and elimination of pain.

Now let's review the information in this chapter:

- **Trauma, osteochondritis dissecans (OCD), and immune-mediated joint disease are the most common causes of osteoarthritis in the hocks of dogs.**
- **Most trauma to the hock occurs when dogs are hit by cars.**
- **Surgery for a hock injury often involves reconstructing the ligaments around the joint.**
- **Your veterinarian may find it difficult to treat OCD of the hock, but fusion of the joint often has an excellent outcome.**
- **Immune-mediated joint diseases (similar to rheumatoid arthritis or lupus in people) are more common in smaller dogs and in smaller joints such as the hock.**
- **Immune-mediated joint disease often causes the joints to break down or collapse.**
- **Your veterinarian can diagnose immune-mediated joint disease by sampling the fluid in the joint. Usually steroids are prescribed.**
- **Joint fusion is used to treat severe collapse of the hock caused by immune joint disease or trauma.**

# PART FOUR

# Dealing with Severe Osteoarthritis

CHAPTER **18**

# MANAGEMENT OF SEVERE OSTEOARTHRITIS

Osteoarthritis in dogs can range in severity from periodic mild discomfort to chronic severe pain. In severe cases it can significantly affect the quality of a dog's life. Dealing with a dog in significant pain can be stressful emotionally and financially.

## Options for Management of Severe Arthritis

- Arthrodesis
- Amputation
- Steroids
- Euthanasia

## Arthrodesis

**Arthrodesis** refers to the fusion of a joint so that it can no longer move. Basically, the surgeon treats the joint

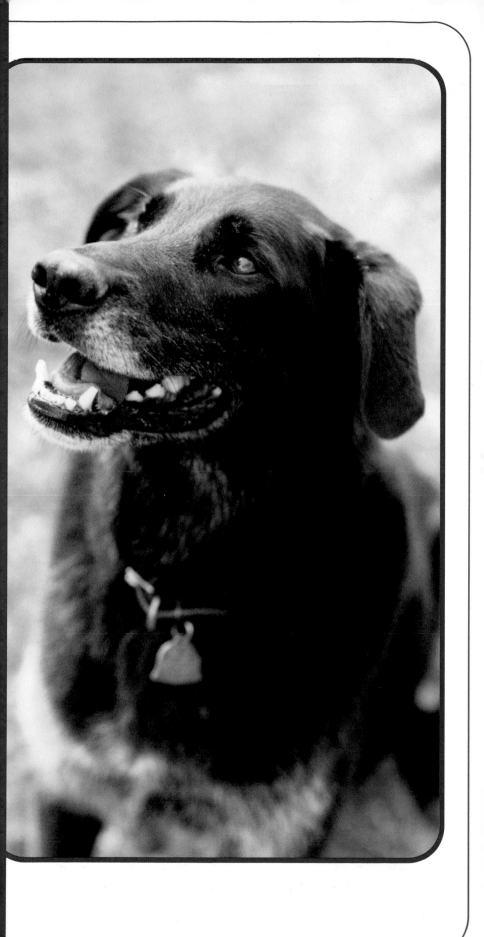

much as one would treat a fracture. The joint is fixed at an angle that is most functional for walking. The cartilage is removed, a bone graft is placed in the joint, and a plate or other fixation device is applied. Often an external splint or cast is applied, because an arthrodesis is usually slower to heal than a typical fracture. Healing times for arthrodesis range from 8 to 16 weeks. Once the arthrodesis is healed, the dog should have no more pain from the joint.

The ability of a dog to function with an arthrodesis depends mainly on the joint that has been fused. Dogs that undergo fusion of the carpus (wrist) or tarsus (**hock** or ankle) can walk, run, and play well. In most cases it is hard for someone without a trained eye to see that a dog has had a fusion of one or more of these joints. Fusion of the elbow, shoulder, or knee does not result in normal function. A dog with a fused elbow, shoulder, or knee will usually stand and walk on the fused limb but may often hold the limb up when running and may hold the limb in an

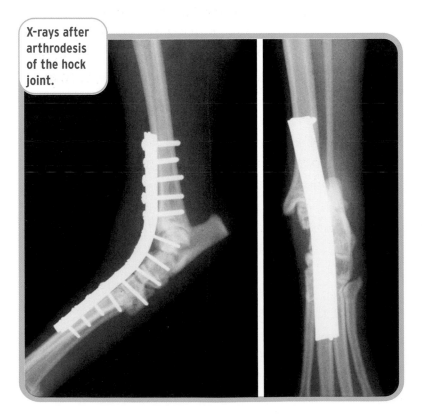

X-rays after arthrodesis of the hock joint.

awkward position when sitting or lying down. The hip joint is never fused because removal of the joint (femoral head and neck **ostectomy**) is a much better option.

Arthrodesis is major surgery that requires an experienced veterinary surgeon and detailed postoperative nursing care by the dog's owner. The end result is generally outstanding for arthrodesis of the **carpus** or tarsus, but function is compromised after arthrodesis of other joints. For this reason, arthrodesis is used for management of only the most severe cases of osteoarthritis. In many cases the osteoarthritis affects more than one leg, so keep this in mind when considering arthrodesis for your dog.

# Amputation

Amputation is the complete removal of a leg. It may be performed at slightly different levels in dogs, but any remaining limb is no longer functional. Prosthetic legs or portions of legs are not usually available for dogs and are not recommended by veterinarians or veterinary surgeons, for several reasons. Prosthetics require significant care, and a dog can't take care of them or tell you when there is a problem related to a prosthetic limb, such as severe skin irritation. Prosthetics are difficult for people to use and even more difficult for dogs to use. We know from experience that a dog will be able to function much better and be much happier with complete removal of a limb than with a prosthetic. And dogs don't seem to care what they look like!

Amputation is often used to treat cancer in a leg but is only rarely used to treat osteoarthritis. This is because in most cases the pain of the osteoarthritis is not so bad that amputation is warranted, or because it can be treated with other methods, such as medication or surgery. If your veterinarian suggests amputation, the status of the other legs must be evaluated. Osteoarthritis often affects more than one joint, and an amputation will increase the load on other limbs.

# Steroids

Steroids are powerful and inexpensive medications that have been used for many years to treat osteoarthritis in dogs; however, these strong drugs also have powerful and dangerous side effects that can be life-threatening. Steroids are routinely used to treat arthritis due to abnormalities of the immune system (**immune-mediated** osteoarthritis) but not for the treatment of common osteoarthritis.

The use of steroids for osteoarthritis is controversial and is usually discouraged by most veterinarians and surgeons. About the only time steroids are recommended for the treatment of osteoarthritis is when a dog has a terminal illness and the veterinarian and the owner are trying to provide some short-term relief.

Steroids for osteoarthritis will usually make the patient feel better for a short time. But the long-term use of steroids actually contributes to the destruction of cartilage, weakens the muscles and other soft tissues, and disturbs the normal hormone function of your dog.

# Euthanasia

At this time, there is no cure for osteoarthritis. Proper medical treatment can dramatically ease the pain of osteoarthritis, as can surgery. Arthrodesis can eliminate the pain of osteoarthritis but may result in abnormal function in some joints. In most cases of osteoarthritis, surgery and medical management can reduce the pain so that the dog can have a high quality of life and function through its natural life span, but in some cases, the pain of osteoarthritis can be so severe and crippling that the veterinarian and the owner simply cannot provide enough pain relief. In these cases, the owner may choose euthanasia. The decision to euthanize a dog should be based on an evaluation of the dog's quality of life, as well as such personal issues as finances and other family situations.

Euthanasia is not a wrong decision, and in most cases the dog has lived a long and wonderful life. In other cases, a young dog may be affected with such severe or extensive joint problems that surgery and medication cannot realistically achieve an acceptable quality of life.

Euthanasia is a difficult personal decision, but veterinarians are there to educate dog owners and support them in the decision that is best for them. Ultimately we are grateful as a profession that we have the humanitarian means to stop severe suffering when other ways are not available.

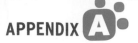

The Body Condition Score, or BCS, is used to judge dogs' body weight relative to their size (see Chapter 5 for a complete explanation). Two scales are available. A scale of 1 to 9 (Nestle Purina) is provided on p. 75. The scale presented in this appendix is based on a scoring of 1 to 5, where 3 is ideal, 1 is severely under-weight, and 5 is severely overweight. These scales are very useful in designing weight-loss diets for over-weight dogs.

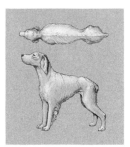

## BCS 1 Emaciated

**What you see**   Obvious ribs, pelvic bones, and spine (backbone), no body fat or muscle mass
**What you feel**   Bones with little covering muscle

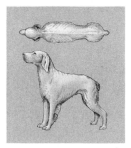

## BCS 2 Thin

**What you see**   Ribs and pelvic bones, but less promi-nent; tips of spine; an "hourglass" waist (looking from above) and a tucked-up abdomen (looking from the side)
**What you feel**   Ribs (and other bones) with no palpable fat, but muscle present

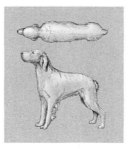

## BCS 3 Moderate

**What you see**   Less prominent hourglass and abdominal tuck

**What you feel**   Ribs, without excess fat covering

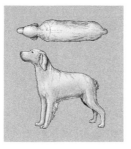

## BCS 4 Stout

**What you see**   General fleshy appearance; hourglass and abdominal tuck hard to see

**What you feel**   Ribs, with difficulty

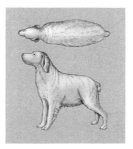

## BCS 5 Obese

**What you see**   Sagging abdomen, large deposits of fat over chest, abdomen, and pelvis

**What you feel**   Nothing (except general flesh)

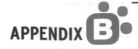

# CANINE BODY WEIGHTS

These body weights have been compiled by the American Kennel Club as rough guidelines for typical body weights for these breeds. Not all dogs of a specific breed will have a healthy weight within the given range.

| Breed | Body Weight (kg) Female | Body Weight (kg) Male | Body Weight (lb) Female | Body Weight (lb) Male |
|---|---|---|---|---|
| Afghan Hound | 23 | 27 | 50 | 60 |
| Airedale Terrier | 19 | 25 | 42 | 55 |
| Akita | 34 | 46 | 75 | 101 |
| Alaskan Malamute | 34 | 57 | 75 | 126 |
| American Cocker Spaniel | 11 | 12.5 | 24 | 28 |
| Australian Cattle Dog | 16 | 20 | 35 | 45 |
| Basset Hound | 18 | 27 | 40 | 60 |
| Beagle | 12 | 14 | 26.5 | 31 |
| Bernese Mountain Dog (Berner Sennenhund) | 4-45 | 50 | 88-100 | 110 |
| Border Collie | 13.5 | 20.5 | 30 | 45 |
| Border Terrier | 5-6.4 | 6-7 | 11.5-14 | 13-15.5 |
| Borzoi | 25-41 | 34-48 | 55-90 | 75-105 |
| Boxer | 24 | 32 | 53 | 70 |

| Breed | Body Weight (kg) | | Body Weight (lb) | |
|---|---|---|---|---|
| | Female | Male | Female | Male |
| Brittany Spaniel | 13.6 | 18 | 30 | 40 |
| Bulldog | 18-23 | 23-25 | 40-50 | 50-55 |
| Bullmastiff | 40-54.5 | 50-59 | 88-120 | 110-130 |
| Calm Terrier | 6 | 7.5 | 13 | 16 |
| Cavalier King Charles Spaniel | 5 | 8 | 10 | 18 |
| Chesapeake Bay Retriever | 25-32 | 29.5-36 | 55-70 | 65-80 |
| Chihuahua | <2.7 | <2.7 | <6 | <6 |
| Chow Chow | 20 | 32 | 44.5 | 70 |
| Collie (Rough And Smooth) | 20-30 | 25-34 | 44-65 | 55-75 |
| Coonhound | | | | |
| Black And Tan Coonhound | 25-34 | 27-36 | 55-75 | 60-80 |
| Redbone Coonhound | 25-34 | 27-36 | 55-75 | 60-80 |
| Miniature Dachshund | 4-5 | 4-5 | 10-11 | 10-11 |
| Standard Dachshund | 7-9 | 12-15 | 16-20 | 25-32 |
| Dalmatian | 22.7 | 27 | 50 | 69.5 |
| Doberman Pinscher | 29 | 40 | 64 | 88 |
| English Setter | 18 | 31.5 | 40 | 70 |
| Flat-Coated Retriever | 25-34 | 25-36 | 55-75 | 55-80 |
| French Bulldog | 8 | 13 | 18 | 29 |
| German Shepherd Dog | 32 | 43 | 70 | 95 |

| Breed | Body Weight (kg) Female | Body Weight (kg) Male | Body Weight (lb) Female | Body Weight (lb) Male |
|---|---|---|---|---|
| Golden Retriever | 25-29.5 | 29.5-34 | 55-65 | 65-75 |
| Great Dane | 55 | 80 | 121 | 176 |
| Greyhound | 27-29.5 | 29.5-32 | 60-65 | 65-70 |
| Irish Setter | 27.2 | 31.7 | 60 | 70 |
| Irish Wolfhound | <48 | <54 | <105 | <120 |
| Keeshond | 25 | 30 | 55 | 66 |
| Labrador Retriever | 25-32 | 29-36 | 55-70 | 65-80 |
| Maltese | 1.8 | 2.7 | 4 | 6 (<7) |
| Mastiff | 75 | 90 | 165 | 198 |
| Miniature Pinscher | 4.5 | 4.5 | 10 | 10 |
| Newfoundland | 50-55 | 60-69 | 110-120 | 132-152 |
| Old English Sheepdog (Bobtail) | 25 | 30 | 55 | 66 |
| Pekingese | 3-5 | 3.6-6.5 | 7-11 | 8-14.3 |
| Pomeranian | 1.5 | 3.2 | 3 | 7 |
| Miniature Poodle | 5 | 5 | 11 | 11 |
| Standard Poodle | 20 | 32 | 44.5 | 70 |
| Pug | 6.5 | 8 | 14 | 18 |
| Rhodesian Ridgeback | 32 | 38.5 | 70 | 85 |
| Rottweiler | 40 | 50 | 88 | 110 |
| Saint Bernard | 50 | 90.5 | 110 | 200 |
| Samoyed | 17-25 | 20-30 | 37-55 | 44-66 |

| Breed | Body Weight (kg) | | Body Weight (lb) | |
|---|---|---|---|---|
| | Female | Male | Female | Male |
| Miniature Schnauzer | 5 | 6.8 | 11 | 15 |
| Scottish Terrier | 8-9.5 | 8.5-10 | 18-21 | 19-22 |
| Shar-Pei | 18 | 25 | 40 | 55 |
| Shih Tzu | 4 | 8 | 9 | 18 |
| Staffordshire Bull Terrier (American) | Na | Na | Na | Na |
| Vizeia (Hungarian Vizsia) | 20 | 30 | 44 | 66 |
| Weimaraner | 32 | 38 | 70 | 85 |
| Pembroke Welsh Corgi | 10-12.7 | 10-13.6 | 22-28 | 22-30 |
| Whippet | 13 | 13 | 28 | 28 |
| Yorkshire Terrier | <3.5 | <3.5 | <8 | <8 |

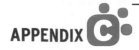

# RESTING ENERGY REQUIREMENTS

The resting energy requirement, or RER, is often used to determine the calorie requirements of dogs on weight-reduction diets. The proper RER to use is that of the target body weight, not the current body weight.

| Target Body Weight | | Resting Energy Requirement (RER) | |
|:---:|:---:|:---:|:---:|
| **Lb** | **Kg** | **RER (kcal/day)** | **80% RER** |
| 1 | 0.5 | 39 | 31.2 |
| 2 | 0.9 | 65 | 52 |
| 3 | 1.4 | 88 | 70.4 |
| 4 | 1.8 | 110 | 88 |
| 5 | 2.3 | 130 | 104 |
| 6 | 2.7 | 149 | 119.2 |
| 7 | 3.2 | 167 | 133.6 |
| 8 | 3.6 | 184 | 147.2 |
| 9 | 4.1 | 201 | 160.8 |
| 10 | 4.5 | 218 | 174.4 |
| 11 | 5.0 | 234 | 187.2 |
| 12 | 5.5 | 250 | 200 |

| Target Body Weight | | Resting Energy Requirement (RER) | |
| --- | --- | --- | --- |
| Lb | Kg | RER (kcal/day) | 80% RER |
| 13 | 5.9 | 265 | 212 |
| 14 | 6.4 | 280 | 224 |
| 15 | 6.8 | 295 | 236 |
| 16 | 7.3 | 310 | 248 |
| 17 | 7.7 | 324 | 259.2 |
| 18 | 8.2 | 339 | 271.2 |
| 19 | 8.6 | 353 | 282.4 |
| 20 | 9.1 | 366 | 292.8 |
| 25 | 11.4 | 433 | 346.4 |
| 30 | 13.6 | 497 | 397.6 |
| 35 | 15.9 | 558 | 446.4 |
| 40 | 18.2 | 616 | 492.8 |
| 45 | 20.5 | 673 | 538.4 |
| 50 | 22.7 | 729 | 583.2 |
| 55 | 25.0 | 783 | 626.4 |
| 60 | 27.3 | 835 | 668 |
| 65 | 29.5 | 887 | 709.6 |
| 70 | 31.8 | 938 | 750.4 |
| 75 | 34.1 | 988 | 790.4 |
| 80 | 36.4 | 1037 | 829.6 |
| 85 | 38.6 | 1085 | 868 |
| 90 | 40.9 | 1132 | 905.6 |

| Target Body Weight | | Resting Energy Requirement (RER) | |
|---|---|---|---|
| Lb | Kg | RER (kcal/day) | 80% RER |
| 95 | 43.2 | 1179 | 943.2 |
| 100 | 45.5 | 1225 | 980 |
| 105 | 47.7 | 1271 | 1016.8 |
| 110 | 50.0 | 1316 | 1052.8 |
| 115 | 52.3 | 1361 | 1088.8 |
| 120 | 54.5 | 1405 | 1124 |
| 125 | 56.8 | 1449 | 1159.2 |
| 130 | 59.1 | 1492 | 1193.6 |
| 135 | 61.4 | 1535 | 1228 |
| 140 | 63.6 | 1577 | 1261.6 |
| 145 | 65.9 | 1619 | 1295.2 |
| 150 | 68.2 | 1661 | 1328.8 |
| 155 | 70.5 | 1702 | 1361.6 |
| 160 | 72.7 | 1743 | 1394.4 |
| 165 | 75.0 | 1784 | 1427.2 |
| 170 | 77.3 | 1824 | 1459.2 |
| 175 | 79.5 | 1864 | 1491.2 |
| 180 | 81.8 | 1904 | 1523.2 |
| 185 | 84.1 | 1944 | 1555.2 |
| 190 | 86.4 | 1983 | 1586.4 |
| 195 | 88.6 | 2022 | 1617.6 |
| 200 | 90.9 | 2061 | 1648.8 |

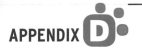

# WEIGHT MANAGEMENT DIETS

| | Hill's Prescription Diet Canine w/d Dry | Hill's Prescription Diet Canine w/d Can | Hill's Prescription Diet Canine r/d Dry | Hill's Prescription Diet Canine r/d Can |
|---|---|---|---|---|
| Calories per cup | 243 | | 220 | |
| Calories per can (size of can) | | 372 | | 296 |
| % Calories from protein | 21 | 18 | 30 | 30 |
| % Calories from fat | 24 | 30 | 25 | 24 |
| % Calories from carbohydrates | 55 | 52 | 45 | 46 |
| Fiber grams/ 1000 kcalories* | 56 | 35 | 78 | 71 |
| Moisture level† | 9% | 74.90% | 9.00% | 75.5 |
| Calories per kilogram food (ME)‡ | 3281 | | 2966 | |

*Fiber is used to increase the bulk of the food and satisfy the dog's appetite. Increased fiber will also increase the amount of feces produced.
†Moisture is used to increase the bulk of the food to increase fullness and satisfy the dog's appetite.
‡Air is used to increase the bulk of the food and make the dog feel full. Fewer calories per kilogram is an indication of more air.

| | Iams Eukanuba Veterinary Diets Optimum Weight Control Dry | Iams Eukanuba Veterinary Diets Restricted-Calorie Dry | Iams Eukanuba Veterinary Diets Restricted-Calorie Can |
|---|---|---|---|
| Calories per cup | 253 | 238 | |
| Calories per can (size of can) | | | 445 (14 oz) |
| % Calories from protein | 29 | 24 | 29 |
| % Calories from fat | 19 | 17 | 19 |
| % Calories from carbohydrates | 52 | 58 | 52 |
| Fiber grams/ 1000 kcalories* | 8 | 5 | 8 |
| Moisture level† | 8.8 | 8.9 | 8.75 |
| Calories per kilogram food (ME) | 3253 | 3648 | |

| Nestle Purina Veterinary Diets OM Overweight Management Dry | Nestle Purina Veterinary Diets OM Overweight Management Can | Royal Canin Veterinary Diet Calorie Control CC 25 Dry | Royal Canin Veterinary Diet Calorie Control CC in Gel Can | Pedigree Weight Maintenance Dry |
|---|---|---|---|---|
| 276 | | 238 | | 240 |
| | 189 (12.5 oz) | | 212 (12.7 oz) | |
| 37 | 55 | 30 | 40 | 28 |
| 16 | 28 | 24 | 54 | 24 |
| 47 | 17 | 46 | 6 | 48 |
| 35 | 78 | 10 | 8 | 5 |
| 10 | 78 | 9 | 84.8 | 8.8 |
| 2726 | | 3590 | | 3679 |

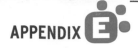

# JOINT MANAGEMENT DIETS

|  | Hill's Prescription Diet Canine j/d Dry | Hill's Prescription Diet Canine j/d Canned |
|---|---|---|
| Calories per cup | 336 | |
| Calories per can (size of can) | | 562 |
| % Calories from protein | 19 | 16 |
| % Calories from fat | 33 | 39 |
| % Calories from carbohydrates | 48 | 44 |
| Omega-6:omega-3 fatty acid ratio* | 0.7:1 | 0.7:1 |
| Total omega-3 fatty acids (EPA and DHA) | | |
| Other supplements | None | None |

*There is still disagreement about which fatty acids are most significant in the dog. The ratios in this table compare linoleic/arachadonic:EPA/DHA

| | Iams Eukanuba Veterinary Diets Adult Plus Dry | Iams Eukanuba Veterinary Diets Senior Plus Dry | Nestle Purina Veterinary Diets JM Joint Mobility Dry | Waltham Royal Canin Veterinary Diet Mobility Support JS 21 Dry |
|---|---|---|---|---|
| | 379 | 358 | 351 | 271 |
| | 24 | 28 | 30 | 25 |
| | 33 | 27 | 30 | 24 |
| | 43 | 45 | 40 | 51 |
| | 7.18:1 | 8.6:1 | 1.8:1 | 16.1:1 |
| | 440 mg/ 1000 Kcal | 300 mg/ 1000 kcal | | |
| | Glucosamine (120 mg/ 1000 kcal) | Glucosamine (112 mg/ 1000 kcal) | None | Green lipped (Perna) muscle |
| | Chondroitin (11 mg/1000 kcal) | Chondroitin (11 mg/1000 kcal) | | |

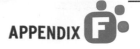

# NONSTEROIDAL ANTI-INFLAMMATORY DRUGS

|  | Aspirin | Rimadyl |
|---|---|---|
| Generic name | Salicylate acid | Carprofen |
| Mechanism of action | Cox 1 and cox 2 inhibitor | Cox 2 > cox 1 |
| Dosage | 10 to 20 mg/kg (5-10 mg/lb) every 12 hours, or prior to activity to prevent pain, or as needed when pain is present | 2 mg/kg (1 mg/lb) twice a day or 4 mg/kg once a day, or as needed for prevention or treatment of pain |
| Side effects | Stomach upset and ulceration, vomiting, anorexia, increased bleeding tendencies, possible liver and kidney effects | Stomach upset, liver disease, possible kidney effects |

| Deramaxx | Etogesic | Metacam | Zubrin |
|---|---|---|---|
| Deracoxib | Etodolac | Meloxicam | Tepoxalin |
| Cox 2 > cox 1 | Cox 2 > cox 1 | Cox 2 > cox 1 | Dual pathway inhibitor |
| 3-4 mg/kg (1.5 to 2 mg/lb) once a day for up to 7 days , 1-2 mg/kg (0.5 to 1 mg/lb) once a day for chronic pain or as needed for prevention or treatment of pain | 10 to 15 mg/kg (5 to 7.5 mg/lb) once a day or as needed for prevention or treatment of pain | 0.1 mg/kg (0.05 mg/lb) once a day (A "loading dose" of 0.2 mg/kg [0.1 mg/lb] may be given on the first day.) | 10 mg/kg (5 mg/lb) once a day (A "loading dose" of 20 mg/kg [10 mg/lb] may be given on the first day.) |
| Stomach upset, liver disease, possible kidney effects | Stomach upset, kidney disease in predisposed dogs, possible liver effects; avoid in dogs with dry eye | Stomach upset, possible colitis, possible kidney and liver effects | Stomach upset, possible colitis, possible kidney and liver effects |

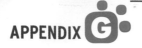

APPENDIX **G**

# OSTEOARTHRITIS MEDICAL MANAGEMENT DIARY

|  | Example | Week ___ | Week ___ | Week ___ |
|---|---|---|---|---|
| Body weight | 45 lbs | | | |
| Diet | X brand light | | | |
| Volume | 1/2 cup twice a day | | | |
| Supplements | X brand 1 gram twice a day | | | |
| Analgesics | X brand 100 mg twice a day | | | |
| Function (running, playing, climbing) | Good (lame after long run) | | | |
| Stiffness | Still stiff in morning | | | |
| Side effects (vomiting, anorexia) | None | | | |

*Copy as needed to create your pet's diary.

# Glossary

**acquired causes**   causes of osteoarthritis resulting from damage to joints or diseases of the joints that develop during the life of the dog. These are different from joint diseases due to genetics.

**acupuncture**   an alternative therapy involving the insertion of small needles into specific points of the body for pain relief or treatment of disease

**aquatic/underwater treadmill**   a treadmill in a small, warm-water pool. The water provides flotation while the treadmill provides movement. The result is low-weight-bearing exercise that is excellent for the treatment of joint disease.

**amputation**   the surgical removal of a limb

**arachidonic acid**   a molecule (fatty acid) in the outer shell of most cells. Injury to the cell causes arachidonic acid to break down into chemicals that produce inflammation and pain.

**articular cartilage**   cartilage found in joints that covers the ends of the bones

**arthritis**   progressive degeneration of a joint (or joints) that leads to pain and impaired function

**arthrodesis**   surgical fusion of a joint. The result of arthrodesis is conversion of a joint to solid bone

**arthroplasty**   surgical modification of a joint

**arthroscopy**   surgical treatment of a joint using endoscopy or specialized telescopes

**arthrotomy**   traditional open surgery on a joint

**bilateral**   condition in which both front or both rear limbs are affected

**body condition score (BCS)**   scale used in dogs to gauge body fat, similar to the body mass index for humans

**body mass index (BMI)**   measure of body fat based on height and weight in humans

**bunny hopping**  simultaneous use of both hind limbs in a hopping manner

**carbohydrate**  family of food that includes the starches and fibers

**carpus**  the joint on the front leg of a dog between the foot and the elbow—similar to the wrist in people

**cartilage matrix**  a spongelike material in cartilage that controls the flow of water and gives cartilage its strength and durability

**Cavalletti poles**  poles that can be placed on ground or slightly elevated and used as an obstacle course

**chiropractic**  manipulation and adjustment of the spine and other joints to attempt realignment of these structures to restore normal posture and body alignment

**chondrocytes**  the cells found in cartilage; chondrocytes are primarily responsible for the production of the cartilage matrix.

**chondroitin sulfate**  an important component of the cartilage matrix. Chondroitin sulfate is important for controlling the amount of water and the strength of cartilage. It is the most familiar glycosaminoglycan and is commonly found in nutritional supplements for joint disease.

**chondromalacia**  softening of cartilage, often the first stage of osteoarthritis

**circumduction**  the movement of limbs in an abnormal pattern. In circumduction the dog often swings the legs out instead of moving them straight forward.

**collagen**  protein found in body tissues that strengthens cartilage

**collateral ligaments**  ligaments on either side of a joint that prevent it from bending abnormally from side to side

**computed tomography (CT/cat scan)**  an electronic imaging device used to evaluate fractures and developmental diseases in joints

**congenital/developmental causes**  causes of osteoarthritis resulting from abnormalities in the growth or structure of the joints. Most developmental causes are genetic in origin.

**conservative management**   also termed *medical* or *nonsurgical treatment*. In conservative management of osteoarthritis the choice is made to avoid surgery and use medications and other treatments.

**contracture**   tightening and loss of joint motion due to muscle shortening and scarring of joint capsule

**cranial cruciate ligament (CCL)**   the ligament that prevents the lower bone of the knee from sliding forward abnormally. The CCL is the most commonly injured ligament in the dog.

**crepitus**   a subtle grinding or crackling feeling that occurs when an arthritic joint moves

**cruciate ligaments**   two ligaments found in the knee that prevent abnormal forward and backward sliding of the lower bone of the knee. Tearing of the front or cranial cruciate ligament is one of the most common joint diseases in dogs.

**cyclooxygenase (COX 1 and COX 2)**   chemicals involved in the production of pain and inflammation in osteoarthritis and also involved in the protection of the stomach and kidneys so that they can have both positive and negative effects on the body

**degenerative joint disease**   another term for osteoarthritis.

**diabetes**   a disease in which blood sugar levels are inadequately controlled as a result of the body's failure to produce or respond to insulin

**disuse atrophy**   weakening of muscles due to lack of use

**dysplasia**   abnormal development of a bone or joint

**eburnation**   polishing and hardening of the exposed bone beneath the cartilage in severe osteoarthritis

**effleurage massage**   gliding stroking of the skin along muscle lines to promote circulation

**endoscope**   a small medical telescope used to examine the inside of the body

**fibroblast** cells that produce fibrous tissue or scar tissue

**fibrocartilage** the most common type of cartilage healing; fibrocartilage heals more easily than normal cartilage but is not as durable or smooth.

**fibrosis** thickening and stiffening of the joint capsule caused by formation of scar tissue

**fragmented coronoid process** a bone chip in the elbow caused by elbow dysplasia

**gait** the speed and appearance of the legs and body during movement

**genetic disease** diseases caused by poor genes

**glucosamine** a type of sugar important in the formation of cartilage; found in many nutritional supplements designed to treat diseases of cartilage

**glycosaminoglycans (GAGs)** an important component of the cartilage matrix. GAGs are important for controlling the amount of water and the strength of cartilage. Chondroitin sulfate is the most familiar glycosaminoglycan and is commonly found in nutritional supplements for joint disease.

**goniometer** large protractor used to measure a joint's range of motion

**growth plate/physis** an area of cartilage found inside bones that is responsible for the growth of bone length in puppies

**herbal therapy** use of herbal extracts and plant parts to treat body ailments, including osteoarthritis

**hip hike** increased vertical motion in the gait. A dog with a hip hike will throw his hip up when the painful limb touches the ground.

**hip sway** increased horizontal motion in the gait. A dog with a hip sway will twist his hip forward when the painful limb touches the ground.

**hock** tarsal joint of the hind leg, between the knee and the foot on the back limb

**homeopathy** the administration of very low doses of toxic substances to boost the natural immune system

**hyaline cartilage** the most common type of cartilage in the body

**hyaluronic acid** the major element in joint fluid that provides lubrication and gives the fluid its thick consistency

**hypothyroidism** low secretion of thyroid hormones essential for metabolic rate and processes. Dogs with hypothyroidism often are low in energy and gain weight easily.

**immune-mediated joint disease** disease in which the body begins to produce cells that attack joint tissues. In immune-mediated joint disease the immune system incorrectly recognizes cells in the joint as diseased and dangerous. The body begins to attack its own tissues, causing pain and inflammation.

**incongruence** when the two bones that meet at a joint do not fit together properly due to genetic, developmental, or traumatic causes

**joint fluid** the thick lubricating fluid contained within the joint capsule that allows smooth, pain-free movement

**joint tap** removal of a sample of joint fluid from a joint for laboratory analysis

**lameness** abnormal use of a limb; most commonly recognized as a limp

**ligament** strong, dense tendonlike structure that connects two bones and provides stability to a joint; prevents abnormal motion in a joint that can damage the cartilage

**lupus** joint disease caused by abnormalities of the immune system

**luxation** dislocation of a joint

**magnetic resonance imaging (MRI)** use of a nuclear magnet for the imaging of soft tissue diseases

**meniscus** thick pad of cartilage in the knee that gives stability and cushioning to the joint

**MSM (methylsulfonylmethane)** a derivative of DMSO, an antiinflammatory used in some select human disease conditions

**muscle atrophy**   loss of muscle mass due to lack of use or to diseases of the nerves

**NSAIDS**   nonsteroidal antiinflammatory drugs the most common antiinflammatory and pain-reducing drugs available

**nuclear medicine**   the injection of small radioactive agents into the body to identify diseased tissues or organs

**nutraceutical**   derived from the words "nutrition" and "pharmaceutical"; a nondrug substance administered orally to promote healing.

**obesity**   the development of grossly excessive amounts of body fat and increased bodyweight

**objective**   studies based on accurate measurement versus opinion

**omega-3 fatty acids**   a nutritional substance used to decrease inflammation in osteoarthritis treatment

**opiates**   strong pain medications that are derived from opium poppies, include morphine, butorphanol, and fentanyl; very addictive in humans

**orthopedics**   the field of study that includes joint and bone disease and treatment

**ostectomy**   removal of a section of bone

**osteoarthritis (OA)**   degenerative joint disease (often used interchangeably with "arthritis"); slow, progressive degeneration of a joint

**osteoarthrosis**   another term for osteoarthritis or degenerative joint disease

**osteochondritis dissecans (OCD)**   a disease caused by abnormal cartilage development, leading to formation of a flap of cartilage within a joint

**osteopathy**   any disease of bone

**osteophyte**   small, round proliferations of new bone associated with osteoarthritis

**osteophytosis**   the presence of osteophytes

**osteoporosis**   loss of bone due to disease process

**osteotomy**   cutting of bone

**palpation** examining and manipulating body structures with the hands to detect abnormalities

**patella luxation** a disease in which the knee cap pops out of its normal position

**Perna mussel** a deep sea muscle that is harvested to make nutritional substances to decrease inflammation in the joints

**petrissage massage** kneading and compression of muscle bellies to relieve muscle tension and spasms

**Physioball** large inflated ball used for strengthening and improving coordination

**polysulfated glycosaminoglycans (PGAGs)** an important component of the cartilage matrix. PGAGs are important for controlling the amount of water and the strength of cartilage. PGAGs are available for injection into the muscle or joint to decrease inflammation in the joint and potentially to promote cartilage healing.

**proprioception** the ability of a dog or a person to know where her limbs are without looking

**prostaglandin** a natural body chemical that causes a strong inflammatory reaction but is also needed for normal body functions. Many antiinflammatory drugs try to block prostaglandins

**proteoglycans** an important component of the cartilage matrix responsible for controlling the amount of water and the strength of cartilage

**radiography** the study of images produced by x-rays

**range of motion** the limits of movement of a joint

**resting energy requirement (RER)** the amount of food (in calories per day) required for a less active dog

**rheumatoid arthritis** a disease of the joints caused by abnormalities of the immune system

**salvage surgery** replacement or removal of a severely damaged or diseased joint

**sclerosis** increased hardness and whiteness of bone

**steroids (corticosteroids/cortisone)** powerful drugs that block the destructive process of the body on cartilage in immune-mediated arthritis.

**stifle**   the knee joint in the hind legs of a dog

**subchondral bone**   the bone found beneath cartilage in joints

**subjective**   data based on opinion rather than measurement

**Theraband**   a large elastic band used in strengthening exercises

**therapeutic ultrasound**   use of high-frequency sound wave energy to produce thermal, mechanical, and chemical effects in treated tissues

**ultrasound**   a visualization tool used for evaluating the soft tissues surrounding a joint

**ununited anconeal process**   a growth abnormality of the elbow where two bones that are supposed to fuse together fail to do so

**viscosity**   the "thickness" of a fluid

# Credits

**Page 21**   Millis D, Levine D, Taylor R: *Canine Rehabilitation and Physical Therapy*, St Louis, 2004, Elsevier.

**Page 42**   Buffington C, Holloway C, Abood S: *Manual of Veterinary Dietetics*, St Louis, 2004, Elsevier.

**Page 47**   Millis D, Levine D, Taylor R: *Canine Rehabilitation and Physical Therapy*, St Louis, 2004, Elsevier.

**Page 76**   Buffington C, Holloway C, Abood S: *Manual of Veterinary Dietetics*, St Louis, 2004, Elsevier.

**Page 132**   Millis D, Levine D, Taylor R: *Canine Rehabilitation and Physical Therapy*, St Louis, 2004, Elsevier.

**Page 144**   Millis D, Levine D, Taylor R: *Canine Rehabilitation and Physical Therapy*, St Louis, 2004, Elsevier.

**Page 204**   Battaglia A: *Small Animal Emergency and Critical Care*, St Louis, 2001 Mosby; courtesy of CVM, University of Missouri-Columbia.

# Index

Hind limb. *See* Hock
Hip
  causes of osteoarthritis in, 248
  dislocation of, 45-47
  radiograph of, 250
  rehabilitation program for, 158-159
Hip arthrodesis, 206
Hip dysplasia, 248-259
  bunny hopping in, 21
  characteristics of, 34-37
  diagnosis of, 254
  phases of, 252
  radiograph of, 251, 253, 258, 259
  therapy for, 254
Hip hike, 20
Hip replacement, 202, 258-259
Hip sway, 20
History, patient, 60-61
Hock, 28
  arthrodesis of, 206
  exercises for, 156, 160
  fusion of, 202
  immune-mediated joint disease of, 278
  lameness in, 20
  osteochondritis dissecans of, 274, 277
  radiograph of, 276
  rehabilitation of, 158-160
  trauma to, 278
Holistic therapy, 222
Home physical therapy, 151-157
Homeopathy, 222
Hyaline cartilage, 11, 12
Hyaluronan, 194-196
Hyaluronic acid, 6
Hydrostatic pressure, 142

# I

Ice pack, 137
Ideal weight, 80-81
Immune-mediated joint disease, 6, 48-49
  of hock, 278
  of knee, 273
  steroids for, 188-189
  of wrist, 246-247
Incongruence, joint, 35
Index, body mass, 74
Infection, 47-48
Inflammation, pain caused by, 14-16
Instructions, discharge, 211-214
Intolerance, exercise, 22-23

# J
Joint
  arthroscopic lavage of, 203
  cartilage in, healing of, 11-12

319

Risk
    of nonsteroidal antiinflammatory drugs, 167-170
    with nutritional supplements, 105
Rottweiler, 44
Running, 120

## S

Scan, bone, 68
Scar tissue, 117
Sclerotic bone, 10
Sclerotic cartilage, 64
Score, body condition, 74-76
    ideal body weight and, 81
Screening for genetic disorder, 54-55
Serpentine walking, 155
Seven steps of weight loss program, 87
Severe osteoarthritis, 280-285
    amputation for, 283
    arthrodesis for, 280, 282-283
    euthanasia because of, 284-285
    steroids for, 284
Shopping for healthy puppy, 49-59
Shoulder, 224-231
    causes of osteoarthritis in, 224
    ligament and tendon diseases of, 230
    osteochondritis dissecans of, 225-229
    radiograph of, 226
Shoulder arthrodesis, 206
Shoulder exercises, 160-161
Shoulder joint, cartilage flap in, 38
Sign of osteoarthritis
    behavioral change as, 23
    change in range of motion as, 23-24
    difficulty rising as, 21-22
    exercise intolerance as, 22-23
    lameness as, 20-21
    muscle weakness as, 25-29
Slow walking, 154-155
Soft tissue
    fibrosis of, 117
    types of, 2-3
Spine flexion, 153
Sprained ligament, 2
Stabilization
    of cranial cruciate ligament rupture, 266
    of joint, 201
Stair climbing, 22
Stationary weight-bearing exercise, 152
Steroid, 188-189
    for severe osteoarthritis, 284
Stiffness, 22
Stifle. *See* Knee
Stimulation, electrical, 138
Strategy, weight loss, 86

Triple pelvic osteotomy, 255
Trot, 147
Turnover, bone, 68

## U
Ultrasonography, 67-68
  in physical therapy, 139
Un-united anconeal process, 235-236
Underwater treadmill, 142-143

## V
Vitamin C, 103
Voluntary exercise, controlled, 118

## W
Walk as normal gait, 147
Walking, 119
  slow, 154-155
Warm-up before exercise, 127, 144
Wasting, muscle, 25-29
Water in cartilage, 3-4
Water level and body weight, 141
Water resistance, 142
Weak ligament, 96
Weakness, muscular, 25-29
Weight, ideal, 80-81
Weight-bearing exercise, 158-159, 160-161
Weight management, 72-89
  body condition scoring and, 74-76
  body weight and osteoarthritis, 73
  caloric density and, 83, 85
  calorie requirements and, 81-83
  exercise and, 112-114
  ideal weight in, 80-81
  life expectancy and, 79
  nutrition in, 73-74
  nutritional supplements in, 90-109. *See also* Nutritional
      supplement
  osteoarthritis and, 79-80
  seven steps in, 87
  starting program of, 77-79
  strategies for, 84, 86
  treats and, 87
Weight shifting, 20-21
Wire repair of cranial cruciate ligament rupture, 266
Wrist
  causes of osteoarthritis in, 244
  exercises of, 162
  fusion of, 202
  immune-mediated joint disease of, 246-247
  radiograph of, 246
  trauma to, 244, 246

# X